Susan's Brother

By

James Marinero

"Let us put our minds together and see what life we can
make for our children."

– *Hunkpapa Lakota Sioux Chief, Sitting Bull.*

Fiction

By

James Marinero

Gate of Tears

A near-future techno-thriller blending bio extraction of minerals, the gold standard and the changing world order with the political, military and industrial emergence of China as the world's leading superpower. With much of the story set in the volatile Yemen and Red Sea region, this action-packed novel takes a fascinating look at what might be just around the corner...

Sicilian Channel

A devastating terrorist attack in Malta's Grand Harbour, political assassination and smuggling set the background to this thriller. With a big score to settle, the psychopathic Serbian terrorist Maruška Pavkovic comes head to head with Steve Baldwin...and they are not kissing!

Follow James Marinero

At

http://www.jamesmarinero.blogspot.com

Twitter @jamesmarinero

Facebook: www.facebook.com/james.marinero

www.jamesmarinero.com

A *Singular* Story

from

Ezeebooks UK
Published by Ezeebooks UK
Ezeebooks UK, 3 Murray Street, Llanelli
Carmarthenshire, SA15 1AQ, UK.
www.ezeebooks.co.uk

Susan's Brother
by
James Marinero

2015 Edition

Copyright © 2012-2015 Phil Marks
ISBN-13: 978-0-9568426-5-7

This is a stylised biography based on actual persons and
events, although some names have been changed. Where
possible, verification of facts has been undertaken.
The hard copy version is printed on paper which accords
with UK: Forest Stewardship Council™ (FSC®) Mixed
Credit.
FSC® C084699

James Marinero is a pen name.

CONTENTS

Prologue

"Ted, why is that man shaking?"

"It's because they are pulsing 600 milliamps of current through his brain every six seconds."

"It must be a Tuesday or a Thursday afternoon, then."

For a young boy in an adult mental hospital, days of the week were relatively meaningless. There were more important things to worry about, confined in a ward with very seriously disturbed adult male patients.

Tuesday and Thursday afternoons in the Nightingale wards at Site 'C'.

Another patient, another brain. Inject a relaxant. Shave the patches, apply the gel, attach the electrodes, check the 'dosage' level, set the timers and switch the machine on. Push the start button. Induce a seizure. Write up the notes.

Tuesday and Thursday afternoons.
Week in, week out, rain or shine.
Scientific.
Therapeutic.

Admittedly, Oak House – Site 'C' at St Augustine's in Chartham, near Canterbury, in 1957 - attempted to treat the worst of the worst patients in societal terms (except the criminally insane). But why was a nine year old boy here, with these mental patients? Why did his mother allow this to happen?

*

"And yet, this young man finds fulfilled joy in later years"

Father's Story

Father was born in Broadstairs in 1910. His own father was a 'businessman', the family was stolidly middle class and were Victorians. Men were men, and boys were young men. No crying, no sign of emotions were allowed. A stiff upper lip was to be maintained at all times.

Father had two sisters, Doris and Gwen, but the males of the family enjoyed primacy in that era.

There was never any sign of affection shown between Mother and Father, and Susan's brother was never hugged by his mother - least of all by his father.

Before the World War II, Father had been a navigating officer in the merchant navy until problems with his eyes had required spectacles and led to him being unable to retain his Watchkeeping Certificate.

After having to leave the merchant navy, he had moved to New Zealand to work as an Air Navigation Instructor. With the onset of war, he changed his plans and in 1942 returned to England. Intelligent, experienced and mature, he was seen as being too valuable to serve with short life-expectancy aircrew in Bomber Command (though he did attempt to join up). He was recruited – passed across by the RAF, really – by the British Overseas Airways Corporation ('BOAC'), becoming a Senior Navigating Officer, ferrying diplomats around the world during the war years.

As civilian aircrew during the years of World War II, Susan's father was not involved in direct action, but was nevertheless exposed to significant dangers.

Warring countries respected the neutrality of countries such as Switzerland, Sweden and Portugal. Civilian flights (both British and German) into and out of those countries were untouched. BOAC regularly flew out into and out of Portela in Portugal from/to Whitchurch near Bristol flying diplomats and others approved by the British Government. For other BOAC flights however, there was no question of neutrality and they were fair game from the outbreak of war. As the war progressed further, attacks by Germany on neutral country flights started. Germany justified them on the grounds that the flights carried spies and escaped prisoners. One such attack by a squadron of Junkers JU 88s on flight BOAC 777A killed the actor Leslie Howard and sixteen other people. The BOAC flight crews were very definitely in the front line.

BOAC wartime flights to Moscow were operated using Consolidated Liberators – an American built aircraft. During peak wartime production, factories designed by The Ford Motor Company were producing them at an overall rate of one aircraft every hour. The first survey flight for the UK to Russia route was on 21/22 October 1942 from Prestwick to Bamenskoye (Moscow) direct, with a flying time of 13hrs 9mins. The dangerous route was over Norway, Finland and eastwards from Riga. Six more flights were made to Moscow direct from Prestwick between 4 January and 4 March 1943.

The only flight with a crew list recorded by BOAC was on 21 January 1943. Subsequently, the route was considered too hazardous and on 10 June 1943 regular flights started from RAF Lyneham routed via North Africa, Cairo, Habbaniyh and Astrakhan.

On 9 October 1943 three flights left the UK on this southern route carrying Anthony Eden and other top level government officials. The family believe that Roy flew on these flights, but there are no records to substantiate this.

The Prime Minister, Winston Churchill also flew this route in November 1943 in a Liberator from the UK to Teheran for his meeting with Stalin and Roosevelt. The pilot was a Captain Vanderkloot, though no other public records exist.

Other crew are believed to have included Johnny Johnson (not the wartime Spitfire Ace of the same name) and Joe Roberts, though this has not been possible to verify.

Roy's best friends were Frank Williamson and Valentine Moore. 'Val' was a flight captain with BOAC. Frank was a dozen or so years younger than Roy. Both he and Valentine had tremendous respect for Roy, who was known as 'Robbo' to his friends and colleagues.

Apart from flying the hair-raising secret flights to Russia, Robbo saw little direct action. He and his close friends (some of whom flew with Bomber Command) survived the war, so there was little direct close personal loss to Robbo, as far as is known.

The crew were billeted at 44 deParis Avenue, Bedford, which was a lodging house run by a Mrs. Somers-Vine, with the help of her two daughters, Valerie and Muriel. Before the war, Valerie had worked as an Assistant Matron at a boys' school in Suffolk, but with the onset of war, both daughters had returned home.

The house was large and comfortable, though it needed updating. The electricity supply was provided by one socket in the middle of the living room floor. The limited 'mod-cons' included an old red Goblin *Triumph* model vacuum cleaner, with a very long lead enabling the whole of the three-storey house to be cleaned from that one socket.

For the aircrew, there were three square meals a day when they were in residence, with the meagre wartime rations supplemented by the vegetable patch and the chickens at the bottom of the garden. They were a lively crew, recognising only too well the limited life expectancy they enjoyed. Frank had survived a tour with Bomber Command, and knew how very lucky he was to be alive. Val had flown Spitfires into thunderstorms as part of research into weather conditions, and had once ended up in a field with the remnants of his 'crate' scattered around him, and no memory of the incident.

Between their hazardous transport flights, life was lived to the full extent that wartime England allowed. The tightly-knit aircrew survived the war intact, and continued together at BOAC.

On the day of their first arrival at the boarding house, Robbo told Valentine that he was going to marry Valerie, the younger of the two sisters.

*

Just after the war ended in 1945, Robbo married Valerie Florence Somers-Vine, as he had predicted he would.

Susan was born in 1946, and Susan's brother in December 1947. The convalescent home where they were born was next door at 42 deParis Avenue.

Within 6 months, there was good news for the family. They were to move to Berkhamsted - a pleasant town on the main London to Birmingham railway line and just an hour by car to the new airport on the A4 west of London - Heathrow. In fact, the main line was at the bottom of the road, and steam trains were an almost continuous sight.

The new house was in a quiet 'close' adjacent to a forty acre field to the north, the Grand Union Canal a few hundred yards away to the south, and convenient for the town centre. With a spinney at the bottom of its long garden, complete with vegetable patch, it was the ideal location for aspiring professional couples to raise families.

There was even a phone box just 200 yards from the house so Robbo could keep in touch with aircrew and BOAC flight control.

The builder, Constantine, built good houses, and Robbo had paid for extras – there was even underfelt, under the tiles. The Williams's, down the road, didn't have underfelt. Though they were good houses for the period, the snow still got into the attic when the bitter winter north easterlies were driving the drifts across East Anglia from the North Sea, and down into Hertfordshire.

Robbo bought a car – it was a Vauxhall and the first car in the close. The family were looked up to. Solid, professional, middle class. England was re-building after the war, and entering an unprecedented period of prosperity.

*

Roy Robinson remained a navigating officer with BOAC flying with the fleet flying the Avro York and the Handley Page Hermes aircraft.

Although Roy had no brothers, he was very close to the male aircrew he flew with, in particular Valentine and Frank. Roy and Frank were particularly good friends and regular golfing partners.

Uncle Frank, as Susan's brother came to know him, was a frequent visitor. He would become a close friend of Valerie, Susan's mother, after Roy's death. Although his loyalty to Valerie over-rode any concern he may have had for Susan's brother – he never interceded - his small gift of a pair of ex-RAF headphones opened a doorway for the young boy.

Valentine Moore too, was a frequent visitor to deParis Avenue and later Dell Field Close. Both Valentine and Frank were addressed as 'Uncle' by Susan and her brother.

*

Robbo sometimes forgot that this was a family unit, and not a flight deck of men who had cheated death every day, who followed orders immediately and without question in the common cause of survival and ultimate victory. Now, although it was peacetime, he worked with the same colleagues as he had in wartime. How much was really different in their war-worn minds?

"Boys can't have teddy bears – they're for girls - you'll grow up soft", Robbo would declare.

Susan's brother wanted a teddy bear because he envied the cuddles that Susan enjoyed with their parents. He didn't get cuddles. One of the neighbour's children was a slightly older boy. He had outgrown his teddy bear and although it was well loved and careworn, Susan's brother was thrilled to be given it. 'Ted' could only see through one eye, so he needed a lot more love than other teddy bears. A strong bond was formed, but Father was not best pleased.

For the family, life was pleasant enough, most of the time. There were picnics on Dunstable Downs watching the gliders; netting the springtime tadpoles at Water End on the Grand Union Canal; warm summers and the early autumn walks around the 40 acre field, picking blackberries.

There were typical middle-England Sunday mornings for a young boy, spent watching his father cleaning and maintaining the car whilst listening to the radio in the garage. Then, Mother's call when Granny, Uncle Popper and Aunty Muriel arrived for a Sunday lunch of roast beef. Although rationing of meat would not end for another two years, Robbo knew the right people, and the family ate well. Evenings playing with the clockwork train in front of the fire, the two cats curled up, the parrot muttering on his perch – life was idyllic, halcyon even, but they were limited. In fact, there could not have been more than a couple of those years to remember before disaster struck the family.

And school – well, that was a different matter entirely for a boy not five years old getting to and from school.

Uncle Frank and Aunty Brenda were regular visitors too, as was Val Moore, by now married to Aunty 'Pete'.

*

Ted's Troubles

The man held Ted firmly.

Strangely, the man didn't seem to be visibly angry.

Thump, thump, thump.

Susan's brother heard the noise as Ted's head hit the wall.

He saw the collision between soft matter and plastered brickwork, heard the noise.

"Boys don't have teddy bears, boys don't have teddy bears", Father's commentary continued with the thumping.

It was a lesson to him, a powerful lesson for a boy not yet four years old.

He would not forget it.

He would remember it vividly for the rest of his life.

Afterwards, he took Ted to his bed.

"Why does he do it, Ted?"

"Because he does."

"That's not a reason."

"No."

"Does it hurt?"

"No."

"I hate to see you get beaten in such a way."

"If not beating me, he would find some other way to teach you. That could be worse."

"I think I'd rather be beaten myself than see you hurt."

"It doesn't hurt. Ignore it."

"But I have to watch you, watch your head hit the wall."

"Yes, but that's better than being hurt yourself."

"But Ted, it does hurt."

"Ignore it, I'm only a toy."

"You are not a toy to me, you are my only friend."

"Some girls are nice to me too, not like Susan."

"It's not as simple as it seems to you. Not all girls are the same. You may not have any real friends, but you do have toys. What about that clockwork train set that your father brought you when he came back from one of his flights, and the Dinky toys?"

"I like that. Yes, I do have dinkies, but why does he beat you Ted?"

"Maybe he thinks I should be a girl's toy. Your father may beat me, but he still lets you keep me."

"I'd like some soft toys."

"Dad says no."

"'least I've got you."

"Not only does Susan have soft toys, but she climbs into bed with Mother and Father on Saturdays and Sundays. They never ask me, and I'm younger. They just don't care about me."

*

Breakfast with Father

Every morning when not on flight duty, father ate his breakfast at home, alone at the dining table. It was always 'a full English' - bacon and eggs, toast and marmalade followed by Camp coffee, with the smell of the chicory-flavoured coffee pervading the room.

As Susan's brother was approaching five years of age, his school results were expected from Edgerton Primary, where he attended five and a half days a week. In reality it was probably only a period of about two weeks terrifying anticipation, but those mornings are deeply etched in his memory.

Each morning during that period, he stood silently in the corner as ordered, and watched his father eat breakfast. His mother cooked the breakfast, but father ate alone.

As a member of a flight crew, Roy Robinson's working pattern appeared to a young boy to be highly irregular, with departures and returns at odd hours. His trips varied in length, but he was usually away no more than a few days at a time. However, during those critical two weeks he was at home every day.

"Same again today Ted, always the same. Stand in the corner until the postman comes, then fetch the mail. Prop it against the toast rack. Father is still talking about my school report."

"What report?"

"He's waiting for a letter from the school about my results."

"But you're not five years old."

"Yes, but they write a report about us – I think about how we can read, do sums. I'm not good at that. I'm frightened. What if my report is bad? I'm scared. Father will be angry if my report is bad."

"You can only do your best."

"Maybe my best's not good enough. I don't know when the results will come. I stand there and wait for the letterbox to rattle. It makes me jump when the letters come through the door and land on the mat. I think I might do well in some subjects, but I think Father will be angry anyway."

"Why should he be angry if you've done well?"

"I don't know. Maybe he thinks it will make me try harder, but all it does is frighten me."

*

"Why does Susan always get an orange and I don't get one at all?
"Don't know."

"I think that it's because everyone thinks she's pretty and clever and I'm fat and ugly. No-one will ever want me. Why waste oranges on me? I'll be lucky to get anything at all if my report is bad."

"Don't be daft you've got to have fruit for school. Everyone does."

"Yes, but I'm worried about my marks. Father talks about them every breakfast time – he's been going on for ever about them."

"Can't have been for ever – you only did the tests a few weeks ago."

"S'pose so. I'm scared though."

"You said you did ok with the tests."

"I thought I did, but what if didn't?"

"Wait and see."

"It's just the sound of the letters arriving when I'm standing there in the corner. One day will be bad I know. It's frightening being there with him."

There are those who believe that the way to motivate someone is to frighten them – the 'stick' approach; then there are those who believe in encouragement. Most successful 'coaches' would say that true motivation lies in sparking the desire to succeed in the subject, and that both carrot and stick are rarely necessary if the internal desire exists. Many people remember one particular teacher in their schooling who had the gift of opening their eyes to a subject, but few of us remember enjoying every subject, less still doing well in them.

For a child not yet five years of age, these theories are less than academic. Few children of that age can reason with a high degree of competence – the driving factors are more emotional and instinctual than based on logic.

Certainly, the emotional pressures on the young boy were felt to be overpowering, and the daily expectation of the school report arriving was magnified.

For a man who has just been through a war, where orders were obeyed instantly and unquestioningly (and lives depended on it), motivating a young boy to do well at school may well have been a challenge. How many other post-war families experienced these same issues?

Were paternal expectations too high, or were there other unrecognised reasons for this apparent failure by the very young boy?

*

"That was it. The results were bad. Father was shaking his head and muttering. He said there were nine - 'subjects' - he called them, and I had done well in three, and average in three, whatever that means. Another three subjects were poor he said. I think that's nine – I can't count so well. Then he shook his head again. I could tell he was cross with me. I don't think I did that badly – however I did would not have been good enough for him.

'What are we going to do with you,' he said?

Then he looked at me and shook his head, he just kept shaking his head. Then, he didn't even finish his toast, just got up from the table and left the room, didn't even say anything to Mother. He was very angry. I'm frightened of what might happen."

Ted was silent.

*

Change at Home

"Why can't I go downstairs for breakfast with Father? He'll be cross if I don't go down."

"Because Mother told you to stay in your room."

"Why has Mother gone to the Williams's, Ted?"

"I don't know. Ask Susan."

"No, I'm not doing that. What's wrong, it's still early; it's not even light yet?"

"Maybe Dad's sick – he's been home for a week with headaches."

"Yes, I suppose so."

*

It was 11th February 1953.

Queen Elizabeth II had acceded to the throne just one year previously. This was her first winter as monarch, with the coronation yet to come. The winter had been cold, dismal, and for many people, poisonous.

In London in December 1952, just two months previously, four thousand people had died and over a hundred thousand had been made ill by smog. Subsequent analysis put the actual number of deaths at twelve thousand.

It is still considered to have been the worst air-pollution event in British history – the smog was even apparent indoors, and led a few years later to the Clean Air Act.

On the last day of January, a storm surge in the North Sea resulted in major flooding and more than two thousand deaths around its coasts as sea levels rose more than eighteen feet above normal.

In Berkhamsted, twenty six miles from the City centre, the Robinson family had been safe from that fatal smog and the flooding, but the winter was about to get worse.

*

When Father was at home he usually got up at about 6 am to make tea. That final morning, Mother heard the kettle whistling and went downstairs to find out why Father hadn't turned the gas off, and she found him unconscious on the kitchen floor.

Her scream did not awaken Susan or her son. The ambulance was called at about 6.15 am from the Williams's home at number 21 - they were the nearest neighbours with a phone. Mother ran there to make the call – it was nearer than the telephone box at the end of the street which the Robinsons would normally use.

Father had been at home for a few days suffering with a headache and unfit for flying duty. This morning, he had got up as usual before Mother, to make himself a cup of tea.

Susan and her brother went off to Edgerton School as usual.

Eventually, at 11 am – almost five hours later - the ambulance arrived.

Father was declared dead at 4pm, in the hospital.

Uncle Frank came round with his wife, Brenda to stand by Valerie as she struggled with her grief and shock at the death of her still relatively young husband.

*

A few days later Mother spoke affectionately to both children about Father's death. He had died of a cerebral thrombosis at the age of 42. That was the last occasion on which Mother ever mentioned Father to Susan's brother.

Susan's brother was five years old and did not go to the funeral. There were no visitors after the funeral, but Uncle Frank and Aunty Brenda were on hand to support Valerie.

*

"I miss him, Ted."

"He's in Heaven."

"I do wonder if he really is."

"I was afraid of Father, he wouldn't let me have a teddy bear and he hated you."

"That was his way. He loved you. He did let you have toys. Don't forget that he bought you a train set."

"S'pose so. At least your beatings will stop."

"The beatings didn't hurt. You still have the train set. Dinky toys too, don't forget."

"Yes, but I don't understand anything."

"He's gone to Heaven."

"Why has God taken him?"

"I don't know."

"It makes me want to cry."

"You can't do that. Boys don't cry."

"I know, but Father's not here to tell me if I do."

"He'll see you from Heaven."

"You think so?"

"Yes, he'll see."

*

Robbo's ashes were scattered on the sea off Broadstairs, where he had been born and raised.

*

The effect of Roy's premature death on the family was serious, not only emotionally, but financially. The welfare state was still in its infancy. Roy had not served long enough to accrue any worthwhile benefits, but BOAC paid Father's salary until Easter that year. The house in Dell Field Gardens had been bought for cash, so fortunately there was no mortgage to be serviced. However, there would be no pension from BOAC. The bank sold the car for Mother.

Mother started to look for work as the end of March 1953 brought a major blizzard and widespread disruption to the South of England. The family home was heavily drifted in, and Council workmen came to dig out the Robinsons and their neighbours.

There were some family resources to draw on – Grandmother Somers-Vine was not rich, but she was comfortable. She lived in deParis Avenue with Muriel, her other daughter - Valerie's sister. Muriel was somewhat timid and held the precocious Susan in awe.

Reality hit the family hard, though, and there was only enough money to educate one child privately. The money came from Granny.

Susan was pretty, bright and clever. She told her brother that he was unwanted and ugly. He believed her. Certainly, his educational progress was not what would be expected from a boy of his age and background. But then, his recent report from Edgerton School had been below Father's expectations. Father, though, was no longer with them.

Granny paid for Susan's education at Berkhamsted Girls School, whilst her brother went to Victoria School for five days a week. At Victoria School he began to develop emotional problems. Edgerton is recalled as a 'grotty' school. Victoria was better that Edgerton in many ways, but for Susan's brother it was no improvement – he was being bullied mercilessly and was, internally, desolate.

Mother had to go out to work. Uncle Frank and Aunty Brenda provided her with emotional support as a good friend of her now-dead husband, but never appeared to stand up for Susan's brother.

*

"Mum talks to Susan, but not to me. She never mentions Father's death."

"'P'raps she find it hard to talk about it."

"She hardly talks to me anyway. And Aunty Muriel, she always tells me that I am 'the man of the house, I must look after my mother, she's my responsibility'. What does that all mean? I don't know what to do."

Ted was silent.

"And Uncle Frank and Aunty Brenda, they say nice things to each other when we go out in the car. He calls her 'Love' and 'Dear'. I never heard Father talk to Mother like that."

"Maybe he did when you weren't there."

"Yes, that's probably it."

*

Susan talked to her friends in school about Father's death – in fact it seemed that she talked about nothing else in school for a couple of years, but her brother could not talk to anyone about it.

After the loss of his father the balance of emotional power in the family began to shift. For Susan's brother, life became more difficult, due less to his father's death than to the failure of Susan's emotional maturity to keep pace with her physical growth. Susan's emotional power needs were drawing both on him and on her mother - her needs were paramount – clothes, pocket money, toys – whatever she needed was there for her.

Her brother had a clockwork train set, a few Dinky toys, and Ted. Susan had a bed overflowing with cuddly soft toys, and her brother envied them out of all proportion to their numbers. Those soft toys represented everything that Susan could have and he couldn't. He was five years of age and expected to behave like a man of the times. He no longer had a father, and his mother appeared to lack any form of emotional link with him.

*

"She's horrid to me, Ted."

"What, who?"

"Susan. She's ignored me until now, hardly spoke to me, didn't play with me. Now she's nasty."

"She misses Father too, you know. A girl needs a father figure."

"But why does she have to call me names?"

"I don't know."

"Everybody thinks I'm fat and ugly and will never make anything of my life."

Ted was silent.

*

At 7 years of age, whilst at Victoria Road School, her brother was enrolled at the Cubs. Attending Cubs required money – there was a four pence weekly fee which his mother gave him.

*

"Where are you going this week then?"

"Same as usual, down to the spinney to play, I'll take my penknife."

"What happens when Mum finds out you're not going to Cubs?"

"Dunno. She won't care anyway. At least I come back with my uniform dirty, so she thinks I've been down to the Scouts Hall and messed about."

"But you're always on your own there, playing by yourself."

"So what? It suits me this way – I'm not paying four pence a week to get picked on. I don't get any pocket money anyway. If Mum can afford the money to send me to Cubs, she can afford to give it to me as pocket money instead."

*

There was one concession to Susan's brother in 23 Dell Field Close. As a boy, he was given the larger of the two bedrooms available for the children. That was the only concession. The big room served only to exaggerate and remind him of the lack of soft toys.

Susan's room was smaller, and her bed was piled with a collection of soft toys.

Ted was the only soft toy that Susan's brother had been permitted, and that had been under protest from his now deceased Father. Father had made his feelings clear with his regular beating of the toy. Was it frustration at some unknown concern, perhaps a childhood problem of his own?

*

Schooldays

Whilst Susan was in her early years at Berkhamsted School for Girls, Susan's brother was attending Victoria Church of England First School, where had started in September 1952.

*

"Ted, why do I have wear my sister's old green blazer to school?"

"Because that's what your mother has given you to wear. She can't afford a blue blazer."

"It's just not fair. Susan gets everything she wants. I don't just get it. I ask her why and her answer is always the same:

"Because you are fat and clumsy, you have no front teeth and you can't read or write. That's why. Get it into your thick head!"

I just hate life, I am so unhappy. Susan is much, much cleverer than me. I can't do anything right – not even catch a ball.

If I go without something then she gets something extra. You think she would be glad to have a bit more, but why does she have to be so nasty to me? I don't understand it."

*

Another Monday.
Susan's brother hated Mondays.
He also hated Tuesdays.
And Wednesdays.
Thursdays and Fridays too.
Saturdays and Sundays were little better.
Susan's brother hated them all.
Equally.

Another Monday – or any other school day - meant being cornered in the playground before school started, wearing a blazer from the hated girls school - a girl's blazer at that.

Cornered in the playground at break, at lunch, afternoon break and yet again after school.

Cornered, taunted, mocked, ridiculed. Abused verbally, endlessly and repeatedly.

Every school day.

Weekends too if he wasn't careful.

He hated waking in the morning to a world that hated him.

Every school morning the same.

Half-terms were worse when Susan was home from boarding.

In or out, Susan's brother couldn't avoid the pain.

He and Ted were walking along the road towards home, have passed at last through the gauntlet of bullying and ridicule for that day, or at least until they got home.

Torture at Victoria School had ended for the day.

School had ended for the day, but not the torture.

He cut a 'Just William' figure in shorts, with his shirt tail hanging out. He was patently unhappy, apparently muttering to himself, kicking stones as he meandered homeward. As usual, he was carrying the hated green school blazer over his arm. If it was raining and he had an overcoat then that helped hide the embarrassment he felt, but today it was a fine spring evening and he had no overcoat.

Over the Grand Union Canal, along Bridgewater Road, past the quiet cul-de-sacs backing onto open country, then Susan's brother turned into Dell Field Close. For Susan's brother, there was no respite at home.

"Ted, please stop them hurting me and give me a blue blazer."

*

Children's Extra-Family Care 1950s

In the 1950's children and adolescents living outside their families (if any) could be in one of several places:

1. Informal adoptive parents (e.g. aunts and uncles)
2. Formal adoptive parents
3. Foster parents
4. Local Authority Children's Homes
5. Special Needs Schools
6. Approved Schools
7. Borstals
8. Runaways with no formal fixed abode.

Victoria Church of England First School

Victoria Church of England First School is an imposing building, red brick, black timbers, dormer windows and a bell tower. Almost Gothic and certainly imposing, designed to impress, perhaps even designed to create a sense of awe in young children. Perhaps even fear. Certainly there have been pupils whose memories of the school are memories of fear.

Victoria School's forerunner was The Bourne School, founded in the eighteenth century by the benefactor Thomas Bourne. Later the Bourne School became the Victoria Church of England School, with the imposing new building. Bourne's birthday is still celebrated every year at the school.

How things have changed in fifty years.
How people have changed.
Perhaps.
Perhaps not.

*

"That was a horrid day."

His eyes were downcast as he trailed his satchel along Bridgwater Road, kicking his toes at the uneven paving stones as he walked home.

"My whole class walking to the Odeon to see the film of the Coronation. All along the High Street, everyone in blue blazers, except me in Susan's old green blazer. It's just not fair. Why can't I be dressed like other boys?"

*

"I hate games! They put me in goal last Wednesday. I'm clumsy, not like all the rest. I can't even catch the ball. Everyone scores against me. How was I supposed to know it's a goal if I carry the ball over the line? No-one told me. I've never played football before, nobody explained the rules to me. Everyone else learned in the park, or with their Dads. And now, when I do save a shot, they laugh, or get angry and hit me."

"That's not true, and some of these boys don't even know their Dads. John's father was killed in that war in Korea."

"Well, brothers or pals then. If I go to the park to play football I get knocked about. They forget about the football and kick me about instead."

*

In 1953, Mother started work at Ashlyns School as a domestic assistant, and had usually arrived home by the time Susan's brother returned from school. She had never worked before, having been brought up helping in her mother's guest house in deParis Avenue, in Bedford. After their marriage, Robbo had provided well for the family, for the seven years of the marriage before his death. The difficulties of the family budget had meant that her initial work was relatively modest, but important to the family, nevertheless.

*

"What do you think, Ted?"

"It's clever, that flashing"

"How do you do it?"

"Battery, bulb and wire."

"The boys in school like it. They call you the Professor."

"Yes, but that's not all they call me. Doesn't stop them hitting me either. I wish I could do something about these teeth. I'm fed up with the bullying."

*

Small children believe all they are told – Father Christmas, the Tooth Fairy, the Bogey Man – until they learn otherwise. Above all they believe their parents, and eventually come to distinguish between 'white lies', and those which have malicious intent.

Normally, this difference is learned within the family, and many are the playground fights that have occurred because one child's parents have told him that there is no Father Christmas and his classmates have taken umbrage.

However, when a child has no father, and little communication with his mother or siblings, then his learning about deceit is much more painful as there is no emotional support when deceit is uncovered; there is no way of pre-empting the usual jokes and half-truths of everyday life which help a child to develop judgement and an understanding that there are grey areas in communication.

Without that support and adult (even peer) feedback, a child's fragile experience and judgement builds slowly and painfully, as there is little coaching in these skills without a solid home background.

*

"I like Mr. Samuel, he gives me cheese."

"Yes, he's funny. And Mr. Booth as well."

"I can't wait for my birthday. A horse of my own. Just like in the cowboys. They promised me they'd get me one."

"Where will you keep it?"

"Don't know. Maybe behind the Close, in the field?"

"Whose field is it?"

"Don't know. I wonder what colour it will be."

"Green."

"No, don't be silly – I meant the horse, not the field."

"Oh."

"I think I'd like a silver one, like the Lone Ranger rides."

"Will you be able to choose?"

"Don't think so. Any colour will be great, though I would really like silver."

"Horses are big. How will you get on?"

"Don't know. A ladder? The Lone Ranger just climbs on, or does a running jump, he's so clever. I want to be a cowboy when I grow up. I don't need to be clever to be a cowboy, and I can wear a mask to cover my face, just like the Lone Ranger. No-one will know I'm ugly that way."

"You're daft. Did you ever see a cowboy in Berkhamsted?"

"No. 'Least, not yet. I'll be the first!"

"Cowboys are in America."

"You can be Tonto."

"But I'm invisible."

"No, you're on my bed, and in my head."

"Do I get a horse?"

"Now you are being daft. You'll have to ride on mine."

"OK. What are you going to call it?"

"Silver. Hi Ho Silver!"

"What if it's brown?"

"Don't know. Browny?"

"Sounds like a girl – y'know, the Brownies?"

"Very funny."

"And what about guns – you'll need two silver ones to be the Lone Ranger. And Tonto carries a rifle."

"I'll ask Uncle Frank. He was in the war, he'll get me some."

"You're daft. The Lone Ranger with guns in Berkhamsted. Hah!"

"Can't wait for my birthday. Come on Tonto. Hi ho Silver!"

"Ok Kemo Sabe"

With that, Susan's brother galloped down the road on his make-believe horse, urging it on with his hand slapping its make-believe rump. He didn't know what happiness was, and those few moments of dreaming about his horse, imagining himself riding down a dry and dusty gulch in the Wild West with Tonto were as near as he got. Just like the Lone Ranger before him, he didn't know that 'Kemo Sabe' means 'wrong brother' in the Comanche language or 'horse's arse' according Gary Larson in a '*Far Side*' cartoon.

*

In 1952, near the bus stop on High Street in Berkhamsted, there was a butcher's shop. On his way to Edgerton School (and in those days it was not unusual for many five year olds to make their own way to school alone), Susan's brother started to call in the butcher's shop. He liked the men behind the counter – Mr. Samuel and Mr. Booth - and they liked him.

*

"Why did they look surprised? I told them it was my birthday today and asked for my horse, just like they promised to give me."

"Find you hankie and stop snivelling, what would Father say?"

"I'm not snivelling! Boys don't cry, I know! But those men lied, they lied to me. Mr. Samuel and Mr. Booth – they lied to me and laughed about it. Why?"

"I told you that you couldn't be the Lone Ranger in Berkhamsted."

"Yes, but I could have had a horse, a small one, just to keep in the field behind the house. They promised me. Promised me! Father tells me never to tell lies. Those men lied to me, and then laughed about it. "

"Father also told you never to cry."

"I can't help it! I'm not crying! They were never going to give me a horse. I hate them. Why do they do it? Why do grown-ups tell lies? I'm never going into that butcher's shop again. I hate them. I hate grown-ups."

"Perhaps they didn't mean any harm."

"I hate them!"

"Come on, wipe your nose – there's the school bell ringing, don't be late."

*

"They are nice, Ted."

Susan's brother was walking home from tea with friends who lived in Hazel Road, just of Swingate Lane, the other side of Berkhamsted.

"Yes, they are nice – I'm not good with words and I don't know what else I can say. They don't have carpets on the floor. And it's damp and cold in the house. Perhaps they can't afford coal for the fire?"

"They are poor."

"How many of them are there?"

"You can count – you know that. There's Tim, his mother and father, and the sisters Catherine and Sally. That's five. And they only have five plates to eat tea from. They have to take turns with the plates when they've got visitors.

"Yes, that's what poor means I suppose. I always get a plate, and one of them has to wait while I eat. I feel awkward about it."

"If they didn't want you there, they wouldn't ask."

"S'pose so."

"You could always ask Tim home for tea."

"I don't think Mum would like that. Tim lives in a council house."

"You never know. Try asking Mum. Anyway, what work does Tim's dad do?"

"I think he works on a building site, some sort of labourer. People think a lot of him, he's nice and genuine, doesn't really earn much though. Well not enough to buy plates and carpets anyway."

"It's hard for them, but doesn't stop them being nice. And Tim's mother keeps the house clean, even though the floors are bare."

"Yes, but poor as they are, Tim still gets a blue blazer to wear to school. I still have to wear that stupid green one. Why?"

"Because that's what Mum says you must wear."

"Why, why, why? We're not as poor as Tim's family. We don't live in a council house."

"Don't get cross, being cross doesn't help."

"I'm not angry, it just that it seems hopeless. A green blazer – a girl's blazer – Susan's OLD blazer. Even the buttons are backwards. It hurts so much."

Tim was not popular in school, so both he and Susan's brother were natural allies. However, Tim's attendance became infrequent and eventually stopped altogether. He was not talked about, and soon forgotten by the other children.

*

Though his mother and teachers did not realise it, some traits were emerging. Somehow, Uncle Frank frequently saw a spark of enquiry in him and one day gave him a set of ex-WD (military surplus) headphones to play with. Now he had light and sound, but it was not enough. His reading skills were still very poor and his writing skills were no better. He was a long way behind his peers. Such children were called 'dunces' or 'planks'.

*

As befitted a Church of England School, there were regular Religious Instruction lessons, and the local vicar would visit weekly to guide the children in their understanding of the Bible, life and religion.

*

"You upset the Vicar. You shouldn't have argued with him."

"Well, how can God be merciful if he took Father away and made me so stupid and ugly?"

"You shouldn't have shouted at him."

"He shouted first, the silly man."

"Don't talk about the Vicar like that."

"Not only that, a real loving God wouldn't have given Susan such a brother as me."

"Don't talk daft."

"It's not daft."

"Anyway, you're in trouble now."

"Can't be much worse anyway. Why are other children always smiling and laughing – at least when they're not crying.

"They are happy when they are smiling and laughing."

"What's happy?"

"Feeling nice."

"I don't understand what that is."

"Try and remember happy days going out with Father in the car, how you felt."

"I can't remember how I felt."

*

One of the teachers at Victoria School was the sister of the headmistress, and her opinion, together with the views of the Vicar and the other staff, led to a meeting about Susan's brother. Action was taken.

The headmistress contacted Mrs. Robinson and explained that the Vicar was of the opinion that Susan's brother was disturbed; that Victoria School could no longer cope with him, and that he would be better at home whilst expert help was sought. In so many words - he wasn't wanted at Victoria Church of England School.

It was made quite clear to Mother that the school could not cope with Susan's brother and that he needed expert help in a more appropriate educational environment where his emotional disturbance could better be managed. This was not an expulsion; it was more like a 'suspension'. The school were very supportive to Mother whilst he was at home and assessment was underway.

His last day in Victoria School was at Easter in 1956.

*

During that time, Mum took him to see a psychologist in Watford, on the advice of the local Education Committee's experts. Disturbed children were relatively few and far between, and most children's homes of the time were geared up to deal orphans and children from 'broken homes'.

With him, Susan's brother took along the ex-RAF headphones that Uncle Frank had given him, and a battery, all concealed in his clothing.

*

"The Professor thought that clicking was strange when he was checking you."

"Yes he was going mental when he heard the headphones clicking through the stetho-wot's it."

"Yeh, dead clever. Mum thought so too – she said you ran rings around him."

"I can hear him now – 'Vot is zat strange clicking'? Zis is very interesting."

"He must be German or something."

"Maybe, definitely not English."

"He wasn't happy with you catching him out like that. He went nuts. He didn't know what to make of you."

"Yeh, but I don't know what he really thought, s'posed to be an expert. He was writing a lot – I'll never be able to write that fast. What are they are going to do with me? What happens to boys like me?"

"Don't know."

*

Eight years old, educationally slow and lacking any real bond with his mother, Susan's brother sank into an emotional pit, into a state of deep depression. He lacked the language to bridge the gap with his mother and explain his feelings – she was remote to him and his non-existent self-esteem, and his father had drummed into him the need to hide any emotion. He was unable to cry, unable to climb up and out of the dark pit into a normal boyhood. There was no helping hand from his mother, no rope or ladder available. He was trapped, and if he tried to climb out, Susan knocked him back down.

And yet, he'd made the Professor in Watford look silly.

The decision that was made by the child care experts of the day, rightly or wrongly, led to a devastating series of events for a lonely and misunderstood boy.

Susan's brother never made it to Ashlyns School; he never made it to any other secondary modern school.

Susan's brother went into special education.

There would be no Eleven Plus examination for him.

Regular qualifications were unnecessary.

At the end of the winter term, he was taken to see Epping House School and joined the school at the start of the summer term in 1956.

Susan's brother had been placed, by well-intentioned adults, into special education, into an experimental school with an unusual but well-meaning approach.

Susan's brother went to a school which failed to provide for his special needs.

*

Berkhamsted Schools

Berkhamsted School for Girls was, and still is, a leading school, both at preparatory and senior levels, taking both boarding and day pupils. In the early 1950's, after the excitement of the Royal Wedding, yet another change of government, and with the strictures of wartime rationing fading into memory, the Berkhamsted girls wore pristine uniforms.

Berkhamsted Boys School is the male equivalent, but the two are entirely separate, in different parts of the town, though each school had a similar ethos, in the broadest sense. At that time, the ideas of boys taking domestic science lessons, or girls playing football were completely unthinkable – the gender stereotypes were rigorously enforced.

Indeed, little had changed even during the war years in Berkhamsted, safely outside the Greater London area, with no strategic bombing targets nearby. Little had changed, other than of course, the loss of some of its young men and women to the war – even some relatively recent pupils of Berkhamsted School.

Pupils came from middle-class stock with fathers who were bank managers and solicitors, print engineers and accountants, civil servants and traffic light engineers, with mothers who helped out at the W.I. - the backbone of England in the post war years. Some fathers - and occasionally, mothers – had been damaged by their wartime trials. Not all damage was visible, but life went on.

At that time, the Berkhamsted School for Girls uniform comprised a green blazer, skirt, knee-length white socks and black shoes. Susan's blazer, and indeed, the rest of her uniform were as smart and clean as anyone else's in the school. No expense was spared to ensure that she received the best education within the family's means, and that she would be given every chance in all respects. Every year or two she had a new blazer. Whatever she needed she received – from tennis racket to hockey stick. She was never short of sweets either – something her young brother could only dream about.

Susan's brother, however, was expected to be a complete disappointment, a failure in life. It seemed to him that he was not wanted.

In contrast, the secondary modern schools - for example Ashlyns – were much tougher environments. The Education Act 1994, also known as the 'Butler Act' (after R.A. Butler, the Conservative politician who shaped it), had redefined post-war schooling. It created the 'secondary modern' schools and raised the school leaving age to 15. They were schools for those who couldn't pass the Eleven Plus exam. Not necessarily because pupils lacked intelligence to pass (though some certainly did), but perhaps because the education system had failed them. Perhaps some were ill-equipped to pass exams with many pupils having few (if any) books at home, little parental support, a poor early education, perhaps even learning difficulties or some other form of what might today be called impairment or even disability.

Some pupils in Ashlyns could not relate to Berkhamsted Girls School or to Berkhamsted Boys School, their pupils and their values. The reverse was certainly true too. Many, if not most, girls from Ashlyns reached puberty a couple of years ahead of their contemporaries at the Girls School – at least, they were wearing makeup and heels when many of the girls from the 'posh' school were wearing their school uniforms even during holiday time. Some would say (and some did) that the girls from the 'posh' school were a class apart.

Generally though, the girls from the two schools disliked each other, and with their male equivalents, Ashlyns versus the Boys' School, that hatred occasionally boiled over into the occasional fight.

The Haves versus the Have-nots, some would have said. Nevertheless, Ashlyns was a good school of its type and enjoyed a reasonable reputation amongst the townspeople.

Nevertheless, the secondary moderns were successful in their time, and turned out many pupils whose crafts ability had shone through in the woodwork, metalwork and other classrooms. Ashlyns Secondary Modern was a successful and highly thought-of such school and turned out many pupils who would in the future provide essential services to the pleasant commuter town of Berkhamsted, pupils who would become valued members of the community, pupils who would work in manufacturing, in the exciting and still relatively new and cherished NHS, in local government, secretarial services and some who would run small businesses of their own - pupils who would be essential to the smooth running of society. Some would go on to become millionaires (if that is a sign of value to society). Even those who would unblock drains would have a valuable part to play. There were successes a-plenty from these vocational schools.

Such craftspeople were in demand in the burgeoning post-war British economy, the economy that would, in 1957, be summed up by the Prime Minister, Harold Macmillan, in his statement:

"Indeed, let us be frank, most of our people have never had it so good."

Seen from Susan's perspective, that might well have been true. However, the operative word in Macmillan's sentence was 'most', and Susan's brother certainly did not experience that sense of well-being, that 'feel-good' factor.

Not all secondary modern pupils would, or could, make a useful contribution or enjoy the 'feel-good' factor.

Some would become casualties of life (joined even by some from Berkhamsted Schools for Girls and Boys in the tumult of the sixties 'sex, drugs and rock'n'roll revolution, some as a result of business failure, addictions and even crime).

Some would be seen as failures for reasons not then understood. The psychological 'radar' for detecting children with Dyslexia or other learning difficulties had not yet been designed or built. Bright or thick, that is all that could be discriminated. Pupils who could not succeed in an academic sense and couldn't build furniture or unblock drains, but had an eye for detail and for sketching or painting might be considered talented artists – in the right environment. The early warning system (or 'radar') for Asperger's Syndrome had not been designed either, so, occasionally another misunderstood pupil fell by the wayside. Bright or thick. Black or white. Grammar or Secondary Modern. But not, in the last analysis, Haves or Have-nots.

The difficulty with 'radar' was that it could not be built until the underlying science was understood, or could at least be formulated to some degree. In the Second World War, understanding of the science underlying radar was led by Great Britain and Robert Watson-Watt, and the success in being the first to build and deploy coastline radar was a key element in winning the Battle of Britain, and of ensuring that the Green Blazers' way of life remained unchanged.

But in Berkhamsted in the early 1950's, the Battle of Britain continued. Berkhamsted School versus the rest. Bright against thick. Green blazers against the rest. Some politically-inclined observers might say that it was the Haves against the Have-nots. Other politically-inclined observers would disagree. They still do today, even though most grammar schools and secondary modern schools have been shunted together in the interests of egalitarianism. Then came mixed ability classes, and then when that notion was shown to be flawed (as it had always had been obvious to many in the teaching profession), then streaming according to ability came full circle.

In time, it would be recognised that other 'radars' – I use it in the sense of a means of early detection - would be needed, but at that time it was not even appreciated that a science was required to start to develop those early warning systems. Dyslexia, Attention Deficit Hyperactivity Disorder, Asperger's Syndrome, Autism and child abuse would require radars, and there wasn't even a science for them at that time but the list would grow as research progressed and more data was collated and analysed. The emerging statistics would indicate the problems and the science would be developed and the radars built. In the meantime, children suffered. Of course, it was no fault of society, or of educational psychologists, the medical profession or anyone else.

In the meantime, life went on in Berkhamsted. A good life for some, but a very difficult and painful life for others.

*

Family Holidays

Between the ages of 3 and 7 years, the young boy and Susan were occasionally sent to a private children's home, on holiday, which they knew as 'Nurse Hill', down in Seaford, near Brighton.

After Father's death, they went only once, and were driven down by Uncle Brian, when Susan's brother was aged six.

The private home was run by a pleasant middle aged lady, who was addressed as Nurse Hill.

*

"I don't want to go."

"It's only two weeks, your mother has to work, and she can't cope with you all the time."

"I hate Nurse Hill, I hate the house, I hate the woman."

"I'm stuck indoors all the time, playing with blocks and stuff. Susan goes out and makes friends. She knows plenty of other children."

"You could go out with her."

"You know I'm ugly and stupid, I can't make friends, and I've had enough of getting jumped and bashed. She won't have anything to do with me – the only time she talks to me is to tell me off for doing something wrong, and then she's really angry. She doesn't even help me when I get bullied."

"Pity John's not here."

"Well he's older."

"But he lives in the Close too."

"Yeh, well he's not here, we come at different times."

"Yeh."

"I'm sick of these wooden blocks."

"Hullo, someone's coming."

*

"Gosh, who was she?"

"Don't know."

"Why did she do that?"

"How should I know?"

"They're different."

"Yeh, haven't got what you've got."

"But why come in like that, lie down and lift her nightie up?"

"Don't know."

"Who was she?"

"Don't know, must be staying here too."

"Must be the same age as us, looks younger than Susan."

"'Prob'ly."

"I haven't seen her before."

*

The following day, Uncle Brian arrived and they drove them back to Berkhamsted. Susan's brother had seen a difference between girls and boys.

*

"Why didn't Father give me the Hornby Double 'O' train set before he died?"

"Don't know, p'raps he was keeping it for Christmas. Mum just said that he bought it. It's been here in the house since he died."

"Why didn't she give it to me before?"

"Search me."

"Maybe she forgot about it."

"P'raps, but I don't think so. Father bought it an' it's been here all that time. I don't know why, but it makes me want to cry."

"Boys don't cry."

"I know, stop keeping on about it!"

*

"I don't get it."

"What?"

"The time. That man said it was 'five and twenty to nine'. What does that mean? Am I late for school?"

"Don't know."

"If it's twenty five to nine, then I know I can get there before the bell and not get a telling off – same if it's eight thirty five, I'll be on time. But five and twenty to nine – what does that mean?"

-36-

"Dunno."

"You left the house at the same time, and you haven't stopped at the butchers."

"No, I am not stopping there ever again!"

"Well it should be alright then."

"I hope so. I don't want another telling off. Five and twenty to nine. What was he talking about? I'll have to think about it."

*

When he was eight years old, Mother bought him a bike from Deerleap garage and taught him to ride it. As was the norm in those days, children would 'go out to play' for hours at a time without any supervision. Riding bicycles, collecting birds eggs and even stealing apples were not unusual pastimes.

His road sense was not the best and he had no 'Cycling Proficiency Certificate'. One day, when crossing the main A41 Aylesbury road, was knocked off his bike. There were no injuries other than a few scrapes. An ambulance happened to pass by and took him home, without a visit to hospital.

"I felt sick in the back of the ambulance wondering about Mother being cross - I thought I was really in for it. I felt like I did when I used to stand there watching father eat his breakfast, waiting for my school report to come with the postman. I hate feeling like that."

"The ambulance men had a job getting you out and into the house."

"I was terrified of Mother and what she'd say."

"Well you're home now."

"Yeh, Mother was nice when I was expecting a real telling-off. I didn't get a hug though. I never do. I'm not sure that she was glad to see me."

*

Maladjusted Children

In 1959, there were 43 hostels in England and Wales for maladjusted children. – *Parliamentary answer by the Minister of Education, April 1959.*

Child Abuse

Quoted from the Crown Prosecution Service Website, retrieved 21st November 2011

'Abuse and neglect are forms of maltreatment of a child. Somebody may abuse or neglect a child by inflicting harm, or by failing to act to prevent harm. Children may be abused in a family or in an institutional or community setting, by those known to them or, more rarely, by a stranger. They may be abused by an adult or adults, or another child or children.'

The Crystal Set

1956 was the year of the Hungarian Revolution.

The Hungarian people were seriously disillusioned with their Communist regime, poor food, lack of life's basics and stultifying propaganda which they rejected entirely, and peacefully. A popular uprising started.

The uprising was escalating out of control, beyond the capability of the Hungarian hardliners to manage with their own resources. There were serious doubts about the reliability of the Hungarian Army, and whether they could be depended upon to shoot their fellow countrymen and control the reaction against the tyranny of the government.

Then, in late October, the Soviet Union started to fulfil a fraternal request from their brothers in the Hungarian Communist Party to quell the popular revolution. This led ultimately to 1,000 Soviet tanks crossing the Hungarian border on 4th November 1956.

The world was on edge, the West impotent and unwilling to get involved beyond grand words. The invasion caused many Western armchair communists to doubt their creed and resign their party memberships.

Many people were fleeing Hungary, and some found their way to the UK and settled there. Some died trying to escape.

In a roundabout way, the Hungarian revolution set Susan's brother on a path which was to save him, though this was before the crisis which led to his sectioning under the Mental Health Act.

*

At the time of the revolution, Mother was working as a domestic assistant in Kilfillan School. The school was a private boys' school run by a Professor Zonafeld. Nick Gynishe was a Hungarian who had fled the country and its Soviet invasion, and come to the UK at 15 years of age. He had found work as an odd-job man at Kilfillan School, and became friends with Susan's mother. Nick had a room in a lodging house off Charles Street, not far from Dell Field Close.

Valerie liked Nick, and he was a frequent visitor to the Robinson home where she offered him a glimpse of 'normal' family life.

Nick took an interest in Susan's brother, who was now living at home and not attending school.

*

Nick made him a simple crystal set (the most primitive of radios), and helped set up an aerial in the garden. These radios comprised no more than half a dozen components plus a earphone. They were so simple that they didn't even require a battery. They were even less sophisticated than those that British secret agents had been using when parachuted into a hostile Europe a dozen years before.

The aerial was a piece of wire 80 feet long which was usually stretched from the bedroom window to the clothesline post at the bottom of the garden.

To a young boy, the set was almost magical.

*

"What's that man speaking, Ted?"

"I can barely hear it through the crackling. It sounds like Chinese to me – maybe it's radio Peking."

"Oh, here's Radio Moscow. Listen."

'The uprising by counter revolutionary forces aided by criminals and traitors has ended and people must carry on with life as normal. They must be ever vigilant of reactionaries and counter-revolutionaries and report any suspicions to the proper authorities. Aided by their Soviet brothers, with hard work and solidarity they will build a glorious and everlasting future for the Party and for Hungary.'

"I don't understand all those long words. It's nonsense."

"Nick knows about the revolution. That's why he came here. Let's ask him to explain. He's good."

"He says I shouldn't believe what Radio Moscow says – it's all lies. How can I believe it if I can't understand it? Why do they use so many long words? Why do people lie? I don't understand the world Ted."

"I don't either."

Tuning the crystal-set (although very limited in scope) radio opened up a world to Susan's brother and was the first crack in the wall imposed by his apparent 'slowness' in school. However, things were to become a lot worse before they would become better.

*

Uncle Valentine and Auntie Pete still called round occasionally to see Valerie, and on one such visit she asked him to repair the electric iron. Watched by Susan's brother, he systematically stripped it down and repaired the internal joint where the old flex had frayed. In those days, the cable sheath was rubber, itself covered by a woven cotton sleeve. The cotton was pleasant to the touch, but water absorbent and not very durable – frayed leads were quite common. He cut and trimmed the cable ends, and refitted them to the internal connections.

However, when he came to reassemble the parts, he had forgotten the order in which he'd removed them, and hadn't laid them out in sequence on the kitchen table. He cursed under his breath – he was being watched by the young lad and making a hash of the reassembly. Seeing his obvious frustration, Susan's brother showed him the order in which the parts should be refitted, exactly.

Uncle Val was amazed - he hadn't until this time seen that there may have been a spark of cleverness in Susan's brother. Uncle Frank had seen it years before when he had given him the old RAF headphones. It was strange that they seemed never to have discussed Robbo's son – at least, not for several years.

Despite his physical clumsiness, this aptitude with mechanical assembly was an ability that would later prove to be a catalyst in his life.

*

"Mum was really cross with you."

"Yeh, but Yatesey shouldn't have split on me like that. We were only messing around. We've never really shot anything with our air pistols. I'd never shoot Yates anyway. That's torn it though, no more playing with Yatesey and our guns in the spinney. Mum's definite about that.

The gun's knackered anyway – the spring was tired when Nick gave it to me, and now Yates is banned from playing with me – a bad influence his father said. Huh! Me? Stupid.

Just because I'm not going to school they seem to think I'm some kind of bad boy."

*

Whenever Nick visited, Mother would greet him with obvious affection and make a big fuss of him. Nick was a very positive influence, and taught Susan's brother the rudiments of boxing. He had introduced him to motorbikes and had given him the air pistol which had led to the problems with Yatesy's parents. Most parents would not have considered this to be a very positive influence. On weekends, they would walk to a café in Berkhamsted where Nick would buy him a Coca Cola.

Despite his being like an older brother, he would not be able to prevent the crisis which was yet to come in the life of the nine year old boy.

*

Epping House School

Following the episode with the headphones, the Austro-German psychologist in Watford had recommended that Susan's brother be sent to a special school which catered for the needs of 'maladjusted' boys. Whether the clicking headphones influenced his recommendation we shall never know.

The term maladjusted was a word of its time. Nowadays in England and Wales, children are not described as maladjusted, but as having special emotional and behavioural needs.

Within Hertfordshire, where Susan's brother lived, the relevant school was 'Epping House Special School'.

It was a residential school near Ware, about 28 miles from the family home in Berkhamsted. Epping House was not a boys' special needs school typical of this period – it was radical and experimental under a recently appointed headmaster who was shaking it up when Susan's brother was sent there early in the summer of 1957.

The main block was an old building on three floors, dating back to the 17th or 18th Century. It was extended in the 1820s by Sir William Horne, who was Solicitor General for a time whilst he owned it. It is, today, a Grade II listed building, with twelve pane sash bay windows on the first floor, and six pane sash windows on the second.

The school's regime (in the broadest sense) was being shaped by the headmaster, Howard Case. His ideas were revolutionary. This school had a serious impact on (or, depending on one's view, failed) Susan's brother. To quote from The Student Voice Handbook:

"In many ways his approach is best understood through the pivotal practice of the Daily Meeting attended by all staff and young people...

...it was here that all significant decisions about how students and staff lived, worked and learned together were taken on a daily basis. The Meeting was chaired by one of the children and normally lasted about an hour...

...The constraining items, such as the Stop or Veto list in which children whose activities were restrained in some way by the will of the Community as expressed in the Meeting, were dealt with first. This was followed by the negotiation of activities that the staff was able to offer in the afternoon and evening, after the 11:00 am–12:30 pm class groups, which the school expected the children to attend. Children were free to choose which activities they wanted to take part in or to offer activities of their own or do nothing at all...

...Then came the allocation of communal work such as sweeping and cleaning and looking after the dogs and cats that had an important role to play in the emotional reparation and development of many of the children in the school."

Of course, from a child's perspective, it was rather different.

*

"I didn't understand why he had to talk about all that stuff, the differences between boys and girls. I know what the difference is."

"After Nurse Hill, yes. Maybe it was just about explaining how boys and girls fit together, how babies are made an' that."

"Yeh. I seem to get called in a lot to talk about this stuff though. We don't do it as a class or anything."

"Don't know."

"And making us run around without clothes on, and have baths with the other boys."

"It's funny alright."

"I don't like having baths with the others. And what's worse is when the cooks and cleaners see me. They laugh – I don't know what's funny about it. I'm the only one who stands out like that. It's almost as bad as being bullied. Either the boys are hitting me or the grown-ups are laughing at my horn. I'm the only one who gets one. Why's that? I'm the youngest too. Why do I have to take my clothes off? They didn't do that in Victoria Park."

Ted was silent.

*

Whether Howard Case's approach to education was influenced by the American Homer Lane's views on the education of children with special needs is not clear. There are obvious similarities between Epping House and the policies and running of Homer Lane's 'Little Commonwealth' at Evershot in Dorset in the years 1913-1918. The 'Little Commonwealth' took in children with criminal records and up to the age of 19 years. Borstals had been established in 1902 – these were more akin to prisons and took in the most serious youth offenders; Approved Schools were established in 1933. These were modelled on the English boarding school, and boarders were drawn from the courts system, offences and other factors deeming this form of open education institution more appropriate than the strict, prison-like regime of Borstals.

Epping House, however, held no such formally convicted young criminals – they were boys who had patent emotional and family problems without a criminal aspect. One or two had had minor skirmishes with the law – usually for stealing food, and such 'crimes' were usually dealt with compassionately.

*

Whilst Susan's brother was a boarder at Epping House, his behaviour worsened considerably, becoming much more hostile both verbally and physically. Medication – tablets – didn't work and his condition intensified.

Some boys cried when they returned to the school from home, and others after there had been a fight. Susan's brother, though, didn't cry. His father's mantra was deeply ingrained:

"Boys don't cry, boys don't cry."

All his angst was internalised, there was no relief, and his unhappiness compounded itself.

*

"Quick, hide!"

The car sped past, up Billet Lane in Berkhamsted. It was now dark and the twenty eight mile walk from Epping House via St Albans had been arduous for a nine year old boy. His feet were sore, and he was tired and very hungry.

"Ok, it's past."

Susan's brother emerged, almost stumbling, from behind the tree where he had hidden as the car approached. He staggered for hiding again as another car's headlights lit his back up, then drove past. He heard the squeal of brakes, and looking up from behind the bush he saw the car reversing. He couldn't make it out in the gloom as it approached and stopped.

"Oh blimey, it's Mr. Gower from the Close."

*

Mum was not at all pleased to see Susan's brother, unexpected at this late hour, or any hour for that matter. The school had not informed her that he had absconded, and she was angry.

Mr. Gower drove him back to the school the next day, having called them late the night before to tell them that Susan's brother was at home.

Back at Epping House, they were concerned for him and he was given medical attention. A twenty eight mile walk would have been more than enough for a fit adult, but this was a nine year-old boy who was far from fit, never played football, and was a poor advertisement for any kind of physical activity, and his feet showed it, and needed treatment.

A few weeks later, he absconded again.

*

"She knew I was coming."

"Yeh, the school must have called her."

"I'm in trouble now. She's cross, the school is cross and I'm in bother. If I run off again then they will not take me back. I hate it here, and I don't want to live at home – I don't even know why I went home. Even home is better than this place."

"Prob'ly"

"I'm just fed up of being a burden to everyone. They all hate me, I'm just a problem. I would be better for them if I was dead."

"Don't say that."

"Well, it's true. I'm just a problem to everyone, they don't want to be bothered, can't be bothered. I might as well be dead."

-46-

Negative thoughts – as with positive thoughts – can reinforce themselves if dwelt on too often. When negative thoughts are constantly amplified by daily contact with others, the consequences can be dreadful, particularly with the absence of any parental love and support.

One night, when he was in bed, a word came into his mind again. It was a word he'd thought about several times recently.

"Ted, Ted, I've thought of something. A way out."

But Ted was still asleep, or not in the mood for talking.

He turned the word over in his mind. He thought about plans, ways, means. At least it was an idea,

Over the next couple of weeks, his resolve hardened as he sunk further into despair.

Ted slept right through this time of planning, did nothing to help shape the idea and the plan. Susan's brother was on his own.

*

Losing Ted

Though Ted' physical embodiment had long ago been left behind or lost – perhaps even thrown out by Mum - Susan's brother could still talk to him. At night, before he went to sleep, with his head on the pillow, when he closed his eyes, Ted was there for him.

There were, though, still some painful images of Ted's head hitting the bedroom wall, but when his eyes were firmly closed, Ted would answer his questions.

He still tried to understand why Ted had been treated so badly.

In time, he realised that he could talk to Ted during the day as well, even with his eyes open. Ted's answers to the repeated questions started to change, to become more refined.

The questions became more specific, and the conversations with Ted less frequent. When they did occur, they were serious.

*

Crisis

"I can't see the point in life."
Ted was silent.
"I don't want to go on living."
Ted was silent.
The boys heard.

"I can't see the point in life."
Ted was silent.
"I don't want to go on living."
Ted was silent.
The staff heard.

Day after day, the word was there is his mind.
"Suicide."
Ted was back.
"Swee what?"
"Suicide, that's what they call it."
"Call what?"
"Killing yourself."
"Where did you hear that?"
"Dunno. Somewhere."
"How do you know it means that then?"
"Dunno, it just does."
"It might mean something else."
"Don't matter, that's what I'm calling it."
"What?"
"Killing myself."
"You're never going to do that!"
"I am, got it all planned, see."
"How?"
"Not telling yet."
"Don't be daft, you're not going to kill yourself."

"Yes I am. Look, nobody wants me, nobody loves me, the boys hit me about and the staff members laugh at me; there's no loving God if there's a God at all, and the vicar thinks I'm disturbed. Dad's dead and Mum doesn't love me. Then Susan says I can't read or write, that I'm ugly and that nobody will ever want me. There's no point, why am I here? I'm going to end my life."

"You can't."

"Why not?"

"It's wrong."

"No-one can stop me. Once I'm dead it won't matter anymore. No one can punish me then. Who cares anyway? No-one, that's who. No-one."

The boys usually slept in dormitories, but Susan's brother was given a room of his own on the first floor. It had been a storeroom, and it was thought better that he should be segregated at night. The teachers and carers were concerned about his condition, which hadn't responded to medication and socialisation at the school, and he was under closer supervision.

"They watch you all the time."

"No."

"OK, well, not when you're asleep."

"That's right."

*

He had been allocated a first floor room of his own for two reasons. One was to keep him away from the other boys at night, and avoid the bullying, and the other reason was to make sure that he couldn't abscond again. The window was too high for him to climb out, down and away.

Tea was at 4 pm in the dining room and there was supper later in the evening. After supper – usually a hot drink and perhaps some cheese on toast at about 8.30 pm, the boys would have a shower and then go to bed.

Susan's brother had been at Epping House through the late winter and spring, without improvement – quite the opposite in fact. It was now mid-summer and getting dark about 9 or 9.30 pm.

His resolve slowly strengthened as his emotional state worsened. Without any emotional support the world made no sense, adults told lies and played tricks on him. He was losing all hope. His conversations with Ted became even more gloomy.

*

"I'm going to commit suicide."

"You don't know what suicide is", said Ted, having found his voice again.

"Yes I do, told you last week. I'm going to end my life."

"You shouldn't. It's wrong and it's against the law? Remember what the Vicar said."

"He was talking rot. There's no point in living. No-one wants me. If there was a God he wouldn't have taken Father and given Susan a fat, ugly brother. There's no God and no point in my life."

"P'raps it'll change, y'know, get better like?"

"How?"

"Dunno."

"Anyway, what are the police going to do when I'm dead? Lock me up? That's a joke. The law is stupid."

"Well, what if it doesn't work, and you end up in hospital. The coppers'll nick you then."

"So, what are they going to do? Can't be worse than now. Then I'll try again."

"Forget it. It's a bad idea, wrong."

"No, it's a way out. I've had enough."

Ted was silent.

Susan's brother turned his face into the pillow. Tears wanted to come, there was pressure behind his eyes, and his lower lip trembled. His eyes were moist, and his heart was hurting. The sobbing was just a breath away, but he closed his eyes tightly and pictured his Father telling him that boys don't cry. Repeatedly he nodded his face hard into the soft feather pillow.

"Boys don't cry, boys don't cry."

He repeated the mantra over and over again, focusing on the words and reinforcing his Dad's stricture, unknowingly reinforcing the programming of his brain with the message, as he had been doing for years.

He was just a young boy, almost ten years old, wanting the misery to end, the huge emptiness of his life to go away; the depression that was consuming his waking hours. Just an end to it, that was all he wanted.

Susan's brother could see an end, could see a way out of the emptiness.

The word suicide was mentioned more frequently, even to other boys in Epping House.

The Headmaster took note and increased the level of supervision. A member of staff was usually stationed on a chair outside the storeroom at night, at least until Susan's brother was asleep

One night, words became actions.

It was just before mid-summer, and the air was redolent with the scents and pollens of the season.

The evening rituals had been observed – it was a warm evening and tomato sandwiches had been made up for supper, with orange juice – there were no hot snacks on warm evenings.

One or two of the boys and staff had hay fever, and supper had been punctuated with their sneezes and sniffles, and the sound of an occasional bumble bee drawn in through the window by the smell of the fresh tomatoes in the kitchen.

In the dormitory, the windows were open to let the fresh air in, and with the light evenings, it took some while for the boys to settle – sunset was after 9 pm, and twilight would persist on this clear evening until after 11 o'clock; the sky would retain some brightness in the north right through the middle of this cloudless night.

Susan's brother was not in the dormitory. He was in the storeroom which served as a temporary bedroom for him – almost a cell, in fact. It was for his own protection, of course, arranged with the best of intentions.

The old window was closed, and the room was stuffy, having been warmed by the sun for most of the afternoon, the door having been shut all day.

The storeroom was only on the first floor, but it was an Edwardian building with high – twelve feet high – ceilings, and copious space under the floors. The building's ground floor itself was raised above the level of the surrounding paved area – there were four steps up into the imposing entrance hall of the building which had been converted from a grand house to an institution designed to educate and make citizens out of problem boys, or 'save them' as the Victorians and the Church would have described its purpose.

After brushing his teeth in the bathroom at the end of the landing, he had gone to bed, strangely not needing to pee. The door was closed. There was no nightly bedtime prayers ritual for this young boy and he went straight to bed. With pyjamas on, a sheet and two blankets, it was hot in bed and he was restless.

*

"Keep still."

"I can't, I'm too hot. I've had enough. Just another horrible day like all the rest. Another belting from the boys, running around without clothes, the cleaners laughing at me, I can't take any more."

The sobs were very close to realisation when his father's mantra came to mind, and as he replayed the events of the day in his mind he turned his head into the pillow.

"Boys don't cry, boys don't cry."

On and on it went.

Then, he took a deep breath and gathered his wits, fighting back the threat of tears. There was no fear in his mind, only blank despair.

Susan's brother slipped quietly out of bed in his pyjamas and crossed the bare and uneven, pine tongue-and-groove flooring to the sash window in his bare feet.

As he pulled the curtains aside, there were tears forming in his eyes – as close as he had ever come to crying since the days of wearing nappies. Father would have been cross if he'd seen the tears in his eyes. But Father wasn't here. God wasn't here. No-one was here.

"Boys don't cry, boys don't cry."

Stiff and encrusted with many coats of fading paint, the old bronze catch on the half-frame of the window at first resisted his feeble, clumsy fingers – they were not the fingers of a boy who played ball games, threw stones or whittled wood, and they struggled with the task; he persisted, his fingers hurt at the unaccustomed effort and then the catch yielded slowly, grudgingly. A struggle that seems to him to last for minutes, was in fact a matter of seconds.

"Boys don't cry, boys don't cry," he recited continuously, the loop repeating, the program in his brain preventing the flood of tears that might have helped to relieve the intolerable weight of his depression. Most children have experienced that moment after a long, deep crying session, when the emotions start to recover with a series of short autonomic breaths and involuntary sounds from inside the top of the mouth – but there was no relief there for Susan's brother, and there never had been.

"Boys don't cry, boys don't cry" he intoned repeatedly as he moved towards escape.

The looping mantra prevented Ted intruding into his consciousness - the program was in control of his emotions. His body, however, was active, but working robotically without conscious direction.

"Boys don't cry, boys don't cry" said his inner voice; outwardly he was an automaton.

With the heels of his palms under the top cross bar of the lower sash, he pushed upwards.

Just as the bronze catch had resisted his fingers, so the sash resisted his shoulders. A short, weak boy, with muscles unused to much exercise, he grunted and heaved. He had never match-wrestled on the grass with other boys, or chopped wood with his father; he had never stacked logs or climbed walls, had never chased wildly across country with a gang of other boys, climbing trees and testing their strength in arm-wrestling matches, racing, long jumping, playing football.

His daily exercise had been as a punch bag.

But though he was a clumsy and frail example of English boyhood, his resolve was now immense, his body running in automatic gear, his mantra keeping intrusive thoughts away, his strength supplied by his hormonal system which had been triggered by the intense but otherwise suppressed emotion of the moment.

The old layers of paint complained at the movement as the window squeaked and squealed and the gap widened. The weak shoulders should have been aching, but the pain pathways were masked by the adrenaline.

A blackbird which had been beaking for supper on the lawn outside was startled as the grip of the paint gave way and the window suddenly slid open. It took flight and fright with its warning call echoing off Epping House's walls and out into the trees beyond the lawn, beyond the paving stones, beyond the window ledge where Susan's brother had finally made the gap in the window big enough for his small body.

He peered over the window ledge.

He didn't stop to measure and analyse. It didn't occur to him. The ground outside was paving stone, flat concrete slabs laid to provide a pathway around the building. It looked like a big drop to a small boy.

It was.

Eighteen feet.

Enough to be fatal.

Few trained adults could have survived the jump without any damage, doubtless even to a paratrooper planning to roll out of the drop onto concrete. Speed at contact would only be about 35 feet per second - 24 miles per hour, though Susan's brother didn't know that. He just expected the fall to kill him. That was his expectation, his intention, his hope.

It was more than enough to kill a nine-year old boy.

At last he had some hope at last, an exit from misery.

He understood the word suicide, understood it was a sin, if indeed there was a God to sin against. He'd argued the case about a merciful God with the Vicar and got into trouble, got into Epping House because of it, got to this window sill because of it - though he didn't see it that way.

He was moving towards a final, lonely fall.

"It's wrong, you mustn't do it."

Ted was back.

The prospect of the eighteen feet fall onto concrete had brought pause to recitation of Dad's mantra, and Ted had broken through the chink in that armour, into his consciousness from that deep, dark space where he resided.

"I can't go on, Ted. I've had enough."

"But what will happen to me?"

"Don't do it."

"There's no point, I must. I've had enough. Can't go on."

"Don't."

Ted may have broken through, but his logic had been over-ridden, his pleas were being ignored.

Susan's brother started sobbing as he hoisted one knee on to the dusty grey paint of the inside window sill, crushing the dead, desiccated flies that had expired there whilst looking for their own way out over years gone by. The mantra came back, then weakened again.

"Boys don't cry...boys don't...boys...

The almost overpowering desire to sob intensified and was pushed away.

At the prospect of death, the deeply entrenched mantra was being superseded by even more powerful programs, programs hard coded by DNA itself, not learned through experience and rote, programs which had protected the human body right through evolution itself.

But the conscious resolve was strong, strong enough to overcome even those from the brain's deepest recesses in this young boy.

With both hands grasping the bottom of the window frame, he pushed off the bedroom floor with his other foot and sat astride the bottom of the window frame, as if in a saddle, ready for a jump. It only required that he lean out and let go. He would probably meet the ground with his head or his right shoulder first, but he wasn't thinking about that. His knuckles were white, his eyes were almost streaming, but he fought the tears back.

"Boys don't cry…boys don't…boys…

The last of the setting sun was red and speckled through the oak trees at the edge of the grounds, shining into his eyes and past him into the storeroom-bedroom. There was a smell of freshly cut grass from the lawns, overlaid with the dusty summer smell of drying hay from the fields beyond the boundary, but he was oblivious to the sights, smells and sounds of a beautiful English summer evening. He was, almost literally, at the end of his tether.

Only seconds had passed since he had climbed out of bed, but time had slowed for him, and it seemed like an age as all the unhappy years of his short life replayed themselves behind the eyes which he had closed in readiness.

Adrenaline, that hormone secreted by the adrenal gland under command from the brain, used by the brain in last-ditch defence of life itself, defence indeed of the brain itself, had given Susan's brother the strength to force that old window open, and give him an exit which would end in his death. What a paradox.

He leaned further outward, and his centre of gravity approached the window-sill median between life and death.

"Stop!" said Ted, too late.

It was irreversible, his centre of gravity was now outside the building and there was nothing Susan's brother could do that would reverse his course, or protect him.

That was it. Over and out he fell, looking forward to nothing beyond escape from his unhappy world.

*

In the corridor outside the storeroom, the staff member on watch duty that night was Mel Perkins. His role at Epping House was that of a 'houseparent' - he is remembered as short, thickset and balding. Slouched in his chair and reading the newspaper, keeping watch on the unhappy boy who had, apparently, never recovered from the death of his father. It was boring duty, as usual, until he heard the creaking, scraping squeal of the century old sash window as it slid open.

He started, and let his well-thumbed copy of the day's Daily Sketch flutter to the floor. With one movement he wrenched the door open and dived across the room to wrap his arms around the disappearing legs of the tortured boy, the boy who was hoping he was one action, one second away from death.

*

The fall stopped before gravity had fully started its work on the young body.

There was a strong firm grip around his legs and shouting. Shouting, who, what? He didn't understand.

No longer falling, he was struggling against some force which was stopping the fall, closing his exit, blocking his escape.

He kicked and struggled, but couldn't overcome the strength that was holding him, slowly pulling him back. Then, as his struggling continued, his centre of gravity was dragged back and crossed the window sill, back into the building.

*

Mel Perkins was shouting for help as he dragged Susan's brother struggling, kicking, wrestling and sobbing, back into the room. His almost-tears turned to anger, and he struggled in rage. Why did Mel stop him? Why couldn't he be left alone to die?

He tried to beat at Mel Perkins's chest with his fists, but he was held firmly, hardly able to move at all.

*

Commitment

All hell broke loose, Mel Perkins was shouting, calling other staff, whilst he held on to and tried to placate the raging boy.

Mr. Case was called.

A doctor was called.

Mum was called.

After speaking to the doctor, Susan's brother was immediately sectioned under the Mental Health Act as a danger to himself.

There was no doubt that the members of staff were concerned. They were caring people and slowly managed to calm him down.

A car was arranged, and two staff accompanied him that late summer evening on the journey to the North Middlesex Hospital. Memories are almost completely absent, his mind was somewhere else.

He was given tablets to sedate him and put in an open ward on the ground floor. All his possessions were taken away as a safety precaution, but the Ward sister allowed him to retain his father's old wartime watch "because it might be of sentimental value". A small kindness, remembered through the lingering fog of those traumatic hours, and across half a century.

The following day, his mother visited.

*

"She cares more about her cats than me."

"How do you know?"

"Obvious. You've seen her looking after them at home. She talks to them. She says nothing to me."

"What about Uncle Frank and Aunty Brenda?"

"They care about Mum – Uncle Frank brought her here himself – but they don't seem to help me."

"But Uncle Frank gave you those headphones. Doesn't that mean something?"

"I suppose so. Mum looked worried."

"She was."

"Brenda's lovely though, she's kind to me. She'd be a lovely mother. Uncle Frank was lucky to find such a nice wife."

"Yes, and the people are very nice here, they care and want to help you."

"Maybe, but it's just a job to them, looking after nutters. The man in the next bed thinks he is Jesus Christ."

"Well, maybe that's better than killing himself. He just wants to be someone other than what he was."

"I just want to be dead. I hate this place. Why do I have to be away from home?"

"Because the nutty professor in Watford thinks you need special help, because they think you miss your father, because you argued with the vicar. That's what they say and they should know. They are experts."

"And they're wrong. At least I'm away from Susan."

It was November 1957, and his tenth birthday was just weeks away.

When Uncle Frank had driven mother to the hospital, he had brought an Airfix kit of a Lancaster Bomber for Susan's brother, who he set about building it. Today, the glue that the Airfix kit needed cannot be sold to minors, because of the danger of solvent abuse. Such abuse was not a concern in 1957, and building the kit was considered therapeutic.

Within a week he had been transferred upstairs to an open adult ward. Many of the patients were traumatised amputees, still fighting or re-living the Second World War or Korea in their minds.

*

"I wonder what it's like not having an arm or a leg?"

"Must be strange. Some of them are really mental."

"They're not all like that – there are some very kind ones too. Johnny Wallace – both hands blown off, yet he smiles and jokes with you.

"I don't think I could be like that if I lost both hands. If I lost both legs I wouldn't want to live. How does he hold his willy, you know, when he pees?"

"Dunno, they pull the curtain round, but he seems to manage,"

"And eating too."

"Listen to yourself! You've got two arms, two legs and all the other bits, and you are in here because you tried to kill yourself."

"Well, maybe all my brain isn't there. I'm not normal - I'm stupid. And fat and ugly."

"Yeh, with two arms and two legs. You're lucky compared to those poor men."

"I'm clumsy too."

"Well, so far the Lancaster Bomber kit looks like the picture on the box – so you seem to be doing that without too many mistakes."

"Just as well it doesn't have to really fly, though."

*

"Jeans, I can't believe it!"

"Well, it is your birthday."

"Yes, but no-one has ever given me clothes that I've liked."

"Somebody cares then, is that what you're saying?"

"S'pose so. Shame about the socks."

"Yes, well it was daft to wash them and put them on the electric fire to dry."

"Maybe, but they shouldn't have melted. The electric fire must have been too hot."

"Fires ARE hot you berk. At least your jeans are ok."

"I'm not letting them out of my sight."

"But they have to go to the laundry, or you'll smell like a tramp."

"They're not going anywhere, I'll wash them myself."

"Just like the socks – you did a good job with those!"

"Jeans don't melt."

"How do you know?"

"Just know."

"You'll look stupid with a hole where your bum should be."

"Now you are being daft."

It was December 1957, his 10th birthday and one not forgotten.

*

The 'North Mid'

"He must be rich."

"He's the head doctor."

"Don't be daft, they're all head doctors here. Nice car though. How does anyone get a car like that?"

"Reading, writing, being clever."

"Is that all it takes?"

"Yeh, of course."

"Well, he needs crazy people to keep him in work. If he cured them all he wouldn't have anybody to fix. He's got to pay for his Aston Martin. A DB2/4 the badge says. Brilliant!"

"That's unfair."

"The world is unfair. There'll always be crazy people for him to try to cure. Maybe there will be new ideas of what crazy is."

"Could be."

"They've got some right nutters in here. Don't know why I'm here though. I'm not mad – or am I? I don't know. It's just that no-one wants me and don't want to be alive."

"Don't talk like that, these people care. The Matron is lovely."

"Yeh, maybe. I still don't understand caring, though. Mother doesn't care, Susan doesn't care. She's not nice but she's got everything. All I have is missing teeth, and I'm clumsy. Nobody will ever want me. Then to top that I can't read or write to save my life, and I don't want to. Save my own life, that is."

"Don't talk like that. You have me too."

"Yes Ted, I have you too, but you can't stop them hitting me."

"Look, there goes Jesus the Second."

"Gosh, yes. I don't think he's getting better though. He still prays for me. Last night he prayed that I'd get the pins to attach the propellers to my Lancaster bomber – didn't work though. God doesn't listen, because there is no God."

"Perhaps you don't pray enough."

"No point, no-one there to listen. I told the Vicar too."

"Yeh, that really led to trouble."

"His own fault. Why won't they let me have pins?"

"'Cos they're dangerous."

"Pins?"

"Yes, you could poke someone's eye with them."

"Me? Never. I hate it here, though, in this place. I just want to be dead."

*

During his four months stay at the North Middlesex Hospital which started in December 1957, Susan's brother spent his daylight hours in the carpentry and craft workshops. He had shown at Epping House that he was adept with his hands. The staff members were caring, considerate of the young boy and genuinely interested in his well-being.

The Matron in particular is remembered for her compassion.

The Lancaster Bomber model was almost complete. However, such planes don't fly without propellers, even in a young boy's mind. He needed pins to attach the four propellers to the Rolls Royce Merlin engines. Prayers from Jesus the Second didn't provide them.

*

One day, there was a palpable sense of excitement at the 'North Mid' and the word was that an eminent Swiss psychiatrist was visiting.

Carl Young - at least, that's how his name sounded to Susan's brother when he was shown into a consulting room and introduced to the pleasant and friendly man behind the doctor's desk.

'Young' his name may have sounded, but he looked old, with wild grey hair. Susan's brother remembers a 'nice old man'. He was someone else who treated the depressed young boy as a human being and not as a problem to be dealt with – even though the boy might have presented an interesting medical case.

The meeting is remembered as being with a kindly and understanding old man – and that in itself was positive for Susan's brother. The belief that somebody really cared about him was not something he encountered often.

Whilst the report of the educational psychologist was being considered, and his immediate future was being determined in meetings and committees elsewhere, Susan's brother was released from the North Middlesex hospital.

There is no recollection of being formally 'released' from commitment, and he wonders whether he was the youngest boy ever to have been sectioned in the United Kingdom.

*

After the 'North Mid' he spent a period at home with his mother whilst his future was being decided elsewhere.

His education was in the form of a few hours a week private tuition. He cycled across Berkhamsted to his lessons, crossing the busy A41 where he had the earlier accident.

This period includes a memory of his first attraction to girls. Although only ten years old, he was smitten by the 16 year- old girl who came out of the private teacher's house every week as he arrived. During his period at home he got to know her – though never her name – and he built a rabbit hutch for her.

During this 'interlude' in his formal schooling and treatment the educational psychologists, psychiatrists and other sundry experts were considering his diagnosis, prognosis and future disposition. Susan's brother was taken by his mother, on two occasions, to the Maudsley Hospital, for further examination.

He was unaware that the prognosis was not optimistic.

*

"Ted, help me. What will they do to me now? Why did they send me there?"

"You are ill, that's why they put you there in the first place."

"Maybe, but am I getting better? It doesn't feel like it, I don't know what's going to happen now. Where will they send me next?"

"We'll just have to wait and see. They would not have let you out if they didn't think it was the right thing for you, so you must be getting better."

*

The Maudsley Hospital

'The Maudsley' as it is known, is a teaching hospital – that is, a hospital where the consultants of the future, already qualified doctors, serve time under eminent consultants, learning more about their chosen specialisation and the intricacies of the human mind. The Maudsley specialises in brains – more specifically the way that brains control, direct and influence the behaviours of the people they inhabit, and manifest those behaviours as individual personalities.

In the psychiatric profession, The Maudsley has enjoyed a long association with the Institute of Psychiatry which grew out of the teaching unit and is part of Kings College, London, and now, a wider association of organisations.

First conceived just after the turn of the 20th Century by Dr. Henry Maudsley, who contributed £40,000 to its construction, it finally opened in 1915 when the Government immediately requisitioned it to treat cases of 'shell shock' (or cowardice, as it was more commonly called in those blinkered days, and which had been the pretext for many courts martial and executions).

It was finally returned to its intended use for civilians in 1923 (and that is not to imply that its wartime work was not valuable).

It also has a linkage with the 'Bethlem (*sic)* Royal Hospital' in Bromley (formerly the St Mary of Bethlehem hospital, which dates back to 1375) – currently they both fall under the management of the South London and Maudsley NHS Trust. The word 'bedlam' is a mediaeval corrupted pronunciation of its name, and came to mean a place of madness and confusion, or more colloquially, 'lunatic asylum'.

Situated in Denmark Hill, Southwark, South London the area has a long association with 'deviant' behaviour. In 'Wild' , Jay Griffiths quotes London's City Fathers as apoplectic with rage about the area, though more so in a licentious sense.

The Maudsley's patient numbers grew rapidly in the 1920's. It soon became apparent that there was a desperate need for a children's unit.

A Child Guidance Clinic was opened in 1928 under the direction of William Moodie as 'The Children's Department'. Teamwork was the central tenet of the approach to diagnosing and treating children: 'psychiatrists to diagnose and to prescribe, psychologists for mental testing, social workers to deal with the environmental side and voluntary workers to observe the activities of the children in the play room' was its stated operational structure.

This was a novel approach, and the importance of research has always been central to the hospital's ethos, as it was to Henry Maudsley in 1907. It retains a worldwide reputation for leading research into mental illness.

An inpatient unit for children was opened in 1947.

Its progress into research made a leap forward in the 1950s when the discipline of Clinical Neuroscience was established, introducing group talking therapies for the treatment of patients suffering specific disorders. Denis Hill propounded a desire to unite the 'two psychiatries' and 'bring psychotherapy into the mainstream of psychiatry'.

*

The first step is the assessment. The assessment has several branches, the branches for a specific patient being chosen according to what has gone before in that patient's history. Perhaps murder. Perhaps attempted suicide. Perhaps on the recommendation of a judge following other deviant behaviour.

Before trial, a defendant would be assessed as to his or her capacity to stand trial, particularly where the circumstances were particularly gruesome or indicative of mental issues.

In 1957, attempted suicide was still a crime. A strange crime, one for which one could not be punished if successful in the full commission of the planned crime. Conspiracy to rob a bank was a crime. Attempting to rob a bank was a crime. Robbing a bank was a crime.

Not so with suicide, though conspiring with another, or assisting, is still a crime today.

Susan's brother was below the age of criminal responsibility, though it very unlikely that any legal action would have been taken – his emotional difficulties were by now well documented.

*

The final, considered diagnosis was that Susan's brother was severely disturbed, and that the condition was probably not curable. It was recommended that he be admitted to a home for disturbed boys, where he would have 24 hour supervision, along with a group of other boys with a variety of behavioural and mental problems. He was expected to spend the rest of his life in mental health institutions.

*

A Day Trip with Mother

"Do we have to go Ted?"

"Yes, Mother says that it's just to look and see if you might like it there."

"I hope that it's better than Epping House."

"Well, at least you'll have the chance to see it first. Mother says that if you don't like it then you can come home."

"I suppose that's fair enough."

"Come on, change your clothes and brush your hair – we have a train to catch."

"If I don't like it, then she says I don't have to stay."

"You already told me that. Where is it?"

"I think near Canterbury."

"Where's that?"

"I don't know, but it's a long train ride."

"I've never been that far on a train."

*

Beech House was situated outside Canterbury. They had taken a train down, with a couple of changes, and then a bus from the railway station.

The psychologists at the Maudsley Hospital had recommended it as appropriate for Susan's brother.

It was a beautiful late spring afternoon, in May 1958, when they arrived at Beech House.

They were met in the administration block by Dr. Turl, a psychiatrist and head clinician, who showed them around.

Beech House was a long narrow building. The front door faced west, with the Charge Nurse's office on the left hand side with the doctor's office. The kitchen was on the right hand side, beyond which was the day room or lounge, with a bar billiards table.

At the end of the building were the toilets and showers, and a padded cell to the left.

As the tour reached the end of the building, Susan's brother excused himself and went into the toilet.

"What do you think?"

"It looks OK, Ted. I like the bar billiards, but I'm not sure about the padded cell. I don't like the look of that."

"And Mr. Vernon, the Head Teacher?"

"He seems nice enough."

"Yes, he does. I think mother likes him."

"I'm worried about the other boys though. They are a lot older than me."

"Wash your hands, we'd better get back."

*

Once the tour of Beech House was over, they went across to Redwood House. This was the new accommodation block, to be opened within a couple of weeks, when the boys sleeping quarters would transfer from Beech House itself. That would enable Beech House to expand its intake. It was after seeing Redwood House that the penny dropped, and Susan's brother realised that he was not going home that day.

*

"Mother tricked me. She said we could go home before deciding."

Ted was silent.

"I don't want to stay. I have no clothes with me, what will I wear? What about my mouse? Who will look after him?"

Susan's brother wanted to cry, but he couldn't. Boys weren't allowed to cry.

Ted was silent.

"She lied to me, she doesn't want me. And Susan's worse. Since I went to the North Mid she's been saying that no-one will want me and no-one will love me. No-one loves me now, so that's no different."

"Yeh, she does seem to be meaner to you."

"She really seems to want hurt me."

"Maybe she's embarrassed about you?"

"I don't understand that, what's embarrassed mean?"

"Dunno, I heard someone say it, can't remember who."

"Her eyes light up when she says those nasty things, it's scary."

*

Susan's brother was signed in to Beech House that same day, and given a bed in the dormitory at Redwood House. He had a small locker and key – all lockers were in the common room – or day room as it was more properly known. Clothes were provided for him.

He was timid and withdrawn, with some physical problems too. There were twelve other boys in Beech House, and Susan's brother was the youngest, the thirteenth child to be placed in Beech House. The bullying started that first night, when he was still suffering from the shock of having been left there by his mother.

*

Beech House

Beech House was the young male wing of St Augustine's Hospital, in Chartham, near Canterbury in Kent, some eighty miles from home at Berkhamsted. So, it could hardly be called local to the family home.

At that time, many young English boys of a similar age were sent away to boarding schools, even further from their family homes. Today, with the greater affluence of the country, even more of the boys (and girls) of England are educated in private boarding schools (i.e. 'public') schools. Even these schools – 'the best educations that money can buy' – were riven with bullying (both emotional and physical) at that time. Although set a generation later, Stephen Fry's autobiography 'Moab was my Washpot' provides a picture of prep school life – and that for a boy who had a loving and stable family home.

The weakest were preyed upon. As Carl Jung said:

'The little world of childhood with its familiar surroundings is a model of the greater world'.

Beech House, though, was no English prep school. Every one of the boys in its care was a patient and suffered with a mental illnesses or emotional disturbance. Their conditions had led many into conflict with the law, family or the wider public.

St Augustine's Hospital was a psychiatric hospital, originally founded as the East Kent County Asylum in 1872. The hospital was incorporated into the National Health Service when it was established in 1948.

The 1845 Lunacy Act made it a legal requirement for counties to provide mental asylum facilities. A site at Chartham near Canterbury was chosen for the second Kent County Asylum (the first was at Margate).

The 'Commissioners in Lunacy' selected the site which satisfied certain basic stipulations, being on elevated ground with a bright vista, near to a town and railway station so that family members could visit easily. Trees were planted around the boundary, as was usual, lest the local population be reminded of its existence. No doubt, the architects would have said that the trees were to provide shelter in the exposed position.

Other, relatively enlightened requirements were for there to be enough land to enable employment and leisure for patients (or inmates as they were known), with segregation from the local population. The site, on a ridge overlooking the valley of the Great Stour, is on the edge of Chartham Downs, an area of Outstanding Natural Beauty. As was usual, the hospital had the full range of facilities expected in a small, self-contained community, including a cricket pitch, shop, chapel and even a cemetery. The hospital was dominated by a huge seven-storey water tower.

In the range of mental institutions in England in the 1950s, Broadmoor, Rampton and Ashworth Hospitals held the 'worst of the worst', the criminally insane, in conditions of the highest security. St Augustine's was on the next tier down.

Security was relatively relaxed, with no sirens to advise the local population in the case of inmate escapes as is the case, for example, in the affluent Berkshire villages surrounding Broadmoor. Generally, the resident patients did not want to escape, and if any did go astray it was usually as a result of confusion. Patients were not considered a danger to others.

*

"I wish I could do something about my teeth. Everybody laughs at them. And then they bully me."

"Your teeth will grow."

"But I look so stupid with this gap in front."

"They'll grow, be patient."

"That bastard charge nurse Oliver just encourages them to laugh at me and bully me."

"He's not a good person."

"What can I do Ted? It's not fair. Oliver just sends us all outside and tells one of the boys to have a go at me. I'm fed up of being knocked about."

"Maybe you should fight back. Nick Gynishe taught you to box remember?"

"I'm frightened. I don't like fighting. I'm really miserable. Father would have known what I should do."

"Maybe he would have told you to fight back. He fought in the war. 'Men should be men' he used to say. Boys too."

"Well, I'm not sure if he killed any Germans or anyone like that. I don't want to kill anyone anyway, I just want them to stop picking on me."

"Well at least Nurse Olive is nice."

"Yes, she's lovely. They have almost the same names – Olive and Oliver, but they are so different."

"Women and men. Different."

"At least not all men are like Oliver."

"Not all women are like Olive."

"Yeh, Mum isn't, for sure."

*

Three weeks later, mother returned. With her she brought his pet mouse and clothes. There was no pocket money, and there would be none. The State would have to provide.

*

"They say they are going to kill Mickey."

"They can't."

"They can – Roger says he will hang Mickey by his tail and poke his eyes out, then cut his tail off. Then they are going to drown him in the toilet and everyone will stab him. Roger said they would become blood brothers that way. Then they will chop him up and feed him to the school cat."

"They won't do that, they're only trying to scare you."

"Roger showed me the knife he said he'll use."

"Tell the Charge Nurse."

"He'll just laugh."

"Tell Dr. Turl."

"I did, and Mr. Wooller too. He says the other boys love Mickey and that they are just joking with me."

"So?"

"I don't believe him."

"What else did he say?"

"He says that the other boys get Mickey out and play with him when I'm not there. He says they love the mouse."

"So, why do the boys say they'll kill Mickey?

Then this morning, Keith said they're going to hang, draw and quarter him, just like they used to do in olden times."

"To mice?"

"No, to people. It's not funny! Stop it!"

"What's drawing and quartering then? Do they, like, get some paper and crayons and draw pictures of him?"

"No! No!"

"So what is it then, maybe it's good?"

"I don't know what it is, but if hanging comes first then it can't be good can it?"

"'S'pose not."

"Then Oliver said they might burn him at the stake. They were all laughing. It was terrible."

"They must be having you on like Mr. Wooller said."

"What do you mean?"

"Y'know, joking, like. Teasing you."

"Why? It's lying isn't it? I don't really understand jokes."

"Cos that's what they do, they tease you, but they tell Mr. Wooller they love the mouse."

"No. Someone must be lying. People always lie to me. Just like those butchers in Berkhamsted."

Ted was silent.

"I'm still worried about Mickey. He's only a mouse, he can't hurt anyone. He lives in a cage. I'm scared stiff that they will hurt him."

"Don't worry. You're lucky that he's in Mr. Wooller's office – no pets allowed here remember. You're getting special treatment. Mr. Wooller is right when he says they love Mickey."

"Huh – they love the mouse? Really? You're joking. Anyway, what's love?"

"Don't start that one again."

"Well, everyone talks about it - not as much as about that sex thing, but still... I don't know what it is. How can someone love a mouse?"

"Don't you love Mickey – isn't that why you are so scared? You have a feeling for him, and when you think of them killing him it makes you feel bad inside, and worry. That's love. How can someone love a teddy bear? How do you feel about me?"

"Nothing, we talk that's all, in secret. You're only in my head."

"Yes, but somewhere, there is the original me, the one who was in your bedroom, lost to you now, probably in a dump somewhere, rotting. How did you feel about me then?"

"Can't remember."

"Don't block it out."

"Not blocking it out."

"Ok. How do you feel about your mouse then? You worry because the others say they'll kill him. That means you feel something."

"I do, that's why I get upset."

"So, that's a feeling for an animal, something inside you."

"Yeh, I s'pose so. Caring though, is that love?"

"It's a start, a good start."

"No-one cares for me. So, no-one loves me. I bet Mum feels nothing inside for me, not like she does for Susan, or I feel for Mickey."

"No, you can care without loving. The teachers here care for you."

"I wish someone loved me, or just cared for me."

"Maybe one day someone will. Go to sleep now."

"'Night."

"'Night."

*

Pets were not allowed, but an exception was made for Mickey, who lived in his cage in Mr. Wooller's office.

Mr. Wooller was the resident psychotherapist, and, as few other people had done, he appeared to be able to see something in the young boy – a spark that could perhaps be kept alight and fanned, before the weight of institutional life extinguished it for ever.

*

Although he received no pocket money from his family, the school provided an allowance of 2/6d a week (half a crown, eight to £1). With this, Susan's brother was able to buy cigarettes – Players or Senior Service. Smoking was openly allowed and three cigarettes a day was sufficient for him.

The cost of the cigarettes was negligible and he began to save some of the weekly allowance.

Wherever young men live together, Pontoon is played – except perhaps in monasteries and the quads of Oxbridge. Beech House was no exception, and the boys played for cigarettes. However, Pontoon was not the only card game played there. Canasta had been devised less than twenty years previously in Uruguay, and was being widely played around the world. Now considered to be a 'classic' card game, it was very popular in Beech House during the time Susan's brother was there.

The bar billiards table was well used too, and it was a game he enjoyed. Despite the need for good hand–eye coordination, and his lack of it, he played often. It was effective physical therapy in its own way, and his coordination gradually improved as the linkage was exercised.

*

Cruelty between the boys was normal. William Golding explored untrammelled boyhood cruelty in 'Lord of the Flies', starting with a relatively healthy and normal group. At Beech House, all the boys were damaged in one way or another and in varying degrees. Group behaviour naturally involved cruelty, both mental and physical. The staff kept it under control, but it was always simmering, and small events triggered the episodes.

Children mimicked what they saw at home, and some of these children had been regular observers of parental fights – murders even - and victims of beatings and other abuse themselves. Such behaviour was part of the way the world worked, in their distorted perception of social interaction. Just as Susan's brother spoke with a

-76-

relatively refined accent copied from his family, so others deployed verbal and physical abuse as part of their unthinking behavioural makeup.

Patrick Mackay, later to become an infamous serial murderer and psychopath, was a patient at Beech House some five years after Susan's brother had left. It has been asserted (Clark and Penycate) that Mackay's problems were due to a drunken, abusive, ex-soldier father who died at a young age, leaving him unable to cope with the loss. Others (e.g. Athens) suggest that such children often manifest their damage in the form of bullying, having at first been victims and learned the behaviour. This takes us back to the earlier quotation of Carl Jung.

The most challenged and damaged children have to be housed and schooled somewhere, and Beech House was such an institution.

Susan's brother was an exceptional patient in many ways, and had not been the victim of, or witness to, any physical abuse at home. His parents' marriage was stable, though he never witnessed any signs of affection between his mother and father; nor did he witness (or does he remember) any signs of strain. His emotional problems were turned inward, and bullying was a behaviour which he was a victim of, never a propagator.

Was this an appropriate educational and, purportedly, caring environment for such a boy?

The boys - patients - at Beech House also reflected the English class system, with their class-social attitudes ('knowing their place') being one of the few things that they had learned at home (beyond, usually, abusive and bullying behaviour).

The pronunciations and manner of speech that Susan's brother used in social interaction had marked him out as being of a different class to the rest of the boys. Susan's brother was considered 'posh'. So, he was either abused or ignored. English social classes didn't mix socially – the boundaries were well defined and closely observed in the early 1950s. Social mobility was a phrase yet to be coined, and certainly not an everyday aspect of life.

Educationally, there was little in the way of structure at Beech House. There were a few nominal lessons in a week, but generally the approach was to let patients follow their own interests. Reading, in particular was strongly encouraged. Unfortunately, not all the boys could read – either because they avoided school, or because they had learning difficulties. At this time, recognition and diagnosis of the forms of dyslexia was in its early stages, even at the research level, and few, if any, teaching staff were aware of it.

Pupils who would today be diagnosed and even 'statemented' were then treated as 'thick'.

*

"Nobody talks to me."

"I do."

"You don't count. I mean the other boys. The only time they say anything is when they make fun of me."

"Mr. Draper the Charge Nurse, Mr. Vernon the head teacher – and his assistant - talk to you. Don't forget the house parents – they talk to you too!"

"That's not the same, you know that. I can't make any friends here. They think I'm different. I talk differently to them - they swear all the time, 'talk common' and say I've got a posh accent. And I never read to the assistant teacher like the others do."

"It's true, you are different."

"Yes, fat and ugly you mean. And posh, with no friends."

"No, you can't help the way you speak, and you are not a criminal or nasty in the way that they are. And you're clever, too. Who else is building a transistor radio?"

"I'm only building one because Mother didn't buy me one and I don't get enough pocket money to buy one myself, not because I'm clever. Susan keeps on about me not being able to read and write, that I'll never get anywhere in life."

"Well, she's wrong. You can read and write – slowly yes, but you're getting better at it. You read magazines, don't forget."

"Maybe, but I hate it here, I really do. It's nearly as bad as Epping House. And the others hate me. I still do stupid things, I know that, but I can't help it.

-78-

Like tonight when I went to eat my cheese on toast, I picked up the cutlery the wrong way round. That set them off again. I can't tell my left from my right. I *must* be stupid. At least I didn't get a thumping though, but I can't help it if I get mixed up. Why can't I remember such a simple thing? Why can't I catch a cricket ball? Why am I so bleeding clumsy? The smallest thing I do wrong seem to start them off. If I wasn't stupid and ham fisted they wouldn't pick on me. They wait for me to do something stupid, and it all starts again."

*

"That was stupid."

"Yes, well…it hasn't happened before, but being here amongst all these bastards who make fun of me and beat me up. It just got too much for me."

"It's hard I know, but the teachers are here to help you. Don't start talking to them like that, like you shouted at the Vicar in Victoria School."

"Look at this place! Not even a bed anyway. How long do you think I'll be in here?"

"Don't know."

"What happens if I want a piss? What do I do then?"

"Just shout I suppose."

"I bet they don't listen. It smells here anyway. I can smell something – pine disinfectant I think, but there's another smell too, very faint. Like – well - old shit or something."

"Can't see a bell or anything."

"No. A padded cell for sure. Rubber walls. Just right for a mad boy."

"You're not mad."

"I did try to kill myself."

"How could I forget! That's not mad anyway, that's ill, and it was months ago."

"Padded cells are so you can't hurt yourself."

"Well, don't do it again."

"Maybe. I wouldn't be at Beech House at all if that Mel Perkins hadn't stopped me jumping. Bastard!"

"Don't blame Mel Perkins, he was only doing his job, caring for you."

"Caring for me? Huh! Is caring a job then, I thought it was something you're supposed to feel?"

"Good question. Maybe you can do both, or maybe there's caring and caring."

"That doesn't make sense."

"Well, look at it this way. You feel for Mickey, and you care for him – give him food, an' that, play with him."

"Yes."

"Well that's one 'caring'. Now, think about Father when he used to clean his car, check the oil, on Sunday mornings, if he was at home. That's 'caring' too, but in a different way."

"Yes, well if he didn't check the oil, then the car would break down."

"That's right. Now, if someone didn't care for you here, give you food and water, then you'd stop working too – kind of break down."

"Ok, I can understand that. But what about my mind – they say I'm severely disturbed."

"Yes, well maybe it's kind of – broken down a bit, you know?"

"Maybe."

"So, you need care."

"I get food and that, you know, but all they seem to do otherwise is talk to me. Where's the care to fix my mind if it's broken a bit, like you say?

"Good question. Ok then, what about a gardener looking after his plants, watering them. They're alive, and he's caring for them."

"But plants don't have minds do they?"

"Don't know, but it makes you think twice about eating cabbage, doesn't it?"

"I don't like cabbage anyway."

"Ok, we're not getting anywhere with this. Look, Mr. Vernon says the others will not kill Mickey, right? The boys say they will. Who do you believe?"

"I don't know who to believe – everyone lies to me all the time. Even the grown-ups."

"The teachers don't lie to you, do they? Or the house parents? Have they ever lied to you?"

"I don't know, maybe they are good liars."

"They don't lie, why should they?"

"Why should the men in the butchers have lied to me?"

"It was a joke."

"I didn't think it was funny. Everyone lies to me or laughs at me. Or hits me."

*

There was no break from the regime, no weekends at home. Sweets and some magazines could be bought in the hospital kiosk and helped to provide some interest and variety. Mr. Draper would occasionally bring magazines in to the school as well – these tended to be outside the normal run of the kiosk fare which was chosen to appeal to the lowest common denominator. The staff maintained hope that they could find a switch in every boy, a switch that would help transform their lives. Generally, it was futile, but they did keep trying. One Monday Mr. Draper brought in a magazine about radios – or wirelesses as they were known then. The magazine contained many long technical words like 'frequency', 'propagation' and 'capacitor'. Susan's brother started reading it though he had no idea what many of these words meant. He had no dictionary, but he devoured the content.

One day, his frustration with the words came to a peak. He asked one of the staff, a Mr. Draper, to explain some of the longer words. The Charge Nurse could see that the lad's interest was palpable and sought to encourage it. Then, the following week, Mr. Draper brought in a copy of 'Practical Wireless' – one of the most widely read 'hobby' magazines for radio enthusiasts.

Susan's brother read the magazine avidly and his interest grew. Though his reading skills were poor – not yet those of a six year-old, his technical radio vocabulary began to expand rapidly. The interest in radio drew him in, and learning to read started to come naturally, without thought. He was no longer being pushed to read, he was being pulled by his interest in the subject.

Mr. Draper developed a particular interest in Susan's brother, offering encouragement and guidance, recognising him as different from the others. Most of those others would, whatever the best-intentioned efforts of the staff and the 'system', change little beyond the physical as they matured. They would be destined to a life of 'failure' on whatever scale that was measured. That, sadly, was the reality, and little has changed since then.

Any lad with potential was supported and encouraged in his individual interests, though it was, on the whole, a Herculean task.

An advertisement in 'Practical Wireless' for a simple '2 transistor radio' became the focus of attention. This radio was a quantum advance on the crystal set - both technically and for his education. It was a huge advance even on the most modern valve radios of the time, which used a lot of power and need a few minutes for the valves to warm up.

He had been given the crystal set by Nick, but this 'tranny' was a kit and had to be assembled – a task requiring a bit more than the glue that his Lancaster Bomber kit had needed. The two transistors provided amplification of the signal, and the set was more versatile, offering access to a wider range of radio stations. The kit had to be assembled by the purchaser, so some tools and a soldering iron would be needed, together with a lot of care and patience.

The kit cost 19/11d – that's 19 shillings and 11 pence (£1), but equivalent to almost £10 in 2011.

Susan's brother ordered the radio kit, posting the order form which he cut out from the magazine. It took two weeks before the kit arrived.

Fortunately, Mr. Draper had a gas soldering iron. These are not the most practical of tools for assembling radios, but this radio was basic (though almost the latest technology at the time) and the gas soldering iron was up to the job. In the late 1950s, practical transistors had been patented only relatively recently. The transistors were the size of a match-head and heat-sensitive, requiring care and delicacy when soldering them to the printed circuit board of the radio. This radio was cutting edge technology for the hobbyist of the day. Small 'pocket' radios were also the seeds from which Sony grew to become a world electronics superpower (though it is said that Sony staff wore shirts with especially large pockets). This small radio was also a fertile seed planted in the mind of Susan's brother.

The kit for the radio arrived, and over a period of a week it was assembled. With Mr. Draper showing him how to use the soldering iron and how to make a good clean and neat soldered joint, Susan's brother completed the project. Patience and a steady hand were important too – something not easy for a young boy.

The radio worked, first time, without any problems.

With the new technology and the advent of widespread access to radio and television stations, the communications revolution began in earnest. In 1964 it would be concisely packaged in the phrase of Marshall McLuhan – "The medium is the message' – still apposite in these 21st Century days of the SMS text message. Britain was entering a period of general prosperity as the world bounced back from the Second World War. Major changes in society were under way, spearheaded by pop music and the emergence of the voice of youth.

In Britain, this was the time of Radio Luxembourg (208 metres Medium wave).

After supper in the evenings, the radios would be turned on in the dormitory, with Jimmy Saville ruling the airwaves. What an unfortunate coincidence.

Almost every one of the other boys had '6 transistor' radios which their parents had bought for them, but Susan's brother had had to make his own from a kit and eke out his allowance for the batteries. Even his modest kit radio was well below the power of those of the other boys but he had built it himself and that was a boost to his confidence. It had other advantages too – with only 2 transistors and an earphone instead of a loudspeaker - a set of batteries lasted him a week. The other boys' radios would use a set of batteries in an evening. So, he was able to stretch his meagre allowance and still have some surplus for sweets and cigarettes.

Music was changing. Rock and Roll from America, Skiffle from England – it was all new and exciting.

*

"Why's Jim here, he's clever isn't he?"

"Yep, he's clever, but I don't think he was clever enough."

"How come?"

"It's those GCEs isn't it."

"What do you mean? Those exams?"

"Well, his parents wanted him to do well, get good results, whatever."

"Not like my Mum you mean. I don't think I'll ever pass any exams. Remember Dad's face when he opened my report from Edgerton? I was scared stiff. I've never forgotten it."

"Yes, your Dad could be scary. I should know."

"Mum wants Susan to do well, but no, she doesn't seem care about me, at least, not so as you'd notice."

"So what about Jim then?"

"The other boys say that his parents, pushed him too hard. Nobody pushes me. Nobody's interested. Nobody cares. Maybe it's a good thing. Jim's parents pushed him too hard and he snapped. A breakdown they call it. Something goes – well, snap - inside, in the head."

"That's why he spends his time painting pictures then?"

"Yep, that's what they call the-rape-you-puticle. 'Least, that's what I think they call it."

"Don't sound good."

"Well, it's only painting."

"You do radios an' stuff. Same kind of thing really. Thera-wotsit."

"Mum's not pushy, she doesn't push Susan either."

"Well, maybe Susan doesn't need pushing. Seems no parents are perfect. It's just that some of us end up in places like this when things go wrong."

"I won't make those mistakes if I ever have kids."

"That's a long way off – you haven't even had your first kiss yet."

"I know, I'm working on it though."

"Who?"

"Not saying."

*

The memories are of a good summer in 1958 in Beech House - sunny summer days, and some form of happiness.

Susan's brother was now ten years old, and was starting to stabilise. The Head Teacher, C. A. Vernon, saw something in the shy and introverted boy, and once, discreetly, took him home for supper.

"What do you think then?"

"About what?"

"Mr. Vernon."

"It was lovely food - his wife is a good cook. Those two tractors though! I'd love to drive one. What does he do with them?"

"It's a smallholding."

"Yeh, so what's that?"

"Dunno. But it looks like he grows stuff – maybe he grows his own food."

"And those batteries – did you see them? Twenty in a row. Just so they can get electric light. I wouldn't like that. He seems happy though. I'd like to be happy, but I don't know how, I can't imagine what it feels like."

*

"It was nice going into Canterbury on the coach."

"Yeh, they took the trouble to come and see me. It was a brilliant day."

"Aunty Gwen is nice."

"Yeh, you can see she cares."

"Did you notice that on the bus, Uncle Norman got me an adult fare?"

"Yes, I'm not a little boy to them."

"She's got a daughter though, Sarah-Jane. Must be a cousin."

"I wonder how many cousins I've got?"

"Well, there's Uncle Norman and Aunty Gwen with Sarah-Jane"

"One"

"There must be more."

"Well I can't remember them. They don't come and see me, if I've got any. Even Mum can hardly be bothered."

*

"Dixon of Dock Green?"

"Yeh. Him."

"That's the copper on the TV?"

"Yeh, that one. Yeh is yeh! Are you deaf?"

"Shhh!"

"Why did he come here?"

"If you sit still and listen, we'll find out."

"I can hardly hear him."

"Shhh!"

"Does he think we are crooks?"

"Don't know, But Mr. Vernon must have asked him to come here."

"Everyone seems to be bored."

"Well he's not a real copper is he, just a TV actor."

"Then why's he dressed like a copper?"

"'Prob'ly his TV uniform."

"Yeh, prob'ly."

"Dunno what the point of it is though."

"Me neither. Can't hear a word."

*

One day, Mother and Susan arrived.

Mother met with Dr. Turl, the psychiatrist at the Children's Unit. After the meeting, the family took a coach into Canterbury for lunch. It was one of those summer's days that Kent is noted for. With a hot breeze blowing in from France, the Garden of England was adding thousands of tons of goodness to the fruit and vegetables in its orchards and farms. The air carried a faint aroma of ripening hops, still at least a month away from harvest.   To most people it would have been a perfect day, but to Susan's brother it was turning into a day of horror. The failed suicide attempt at Epping House was still vivid in his memory, followed by the torment at the 'North Mid' as he struggled with the reality of his failed escape from life.

As the coach drove in towards Canterbury, Mother told him that Beech House was closing for two weeks summer holiday, and that he would be coming home to South Park Gardens.

Then he asked if Susan would be at home during the holiday. Mother told him that of course she would – she would be on holiday too.

He recoiled into the corner of his seat in horror and his words to his mother were instantaneous and vehement. He would not spend a holiday at home with Susan. He would run away before doing that.

Then he closed his eyes, shaking his head and turning inward.

"I don't want to go home, Ted."

"You have to. There are two weeks summer holiday, Beech House is closing down for the summer holiday. Even the boys in Ashlyns get seven weeks off.

"I don't want to go home. I want to stay here."

"You must go. Beech House will be closed."

"Susan will be at home – it's her holiday too – I couldn't stand it. I'll run away if I have to go home and Susan is there. There must be something that they can do, somewhere else I can go; not back to Epping House though."

The conversation continued in his head, in his own world. Lunch in Canterbury was a strained affair, and when Susan's brother found his voice, he was still unequivocal as he spoke to his mother. He would not be persuaded.

As the coach drove back to Beech House, his Mother looked at him, not understanding, failing to get any response out of him. His sister was completely disinterested.

He was in his own world.

He would not spend a holiday at home with Susan.

There was no normal brother/sister connection, support or protectiveness. He was an embarrassment to his sister and the dislike between them was strong and mutual. He felt it deeply.

*

As they climbed off the coach, he was silent and withdrawn. Susan stayed on the coach, whilst mother accompanied him to Dr. Turl's office.

*

-87-

At the earlier meeting with Mother, Dr. Turl had explained the predicament - the unit, Beech House, was closing for the summer holiday, as it did every year.

Mother explained to Dr. Turl that Susan's brother did not want to go home for the holidays - he was adamant, and she was concerned about what might happen if he did.

There was only one solution that Dr. Turl could suggest.

The ten year old boy would have to be transferred to Oak House, at St Augustine's. To the Adult Unit.

Something must have been lost in the message, because no normal mother would surely have contemplated the Adult Unit as a solution to the problem. Did she question Dr. Turl about the implications? And what of Dr. Turl? Surely he would have appreciated that it was not an appropriate solution?

Looking back, we cannot know the details, but one thing was certain. For Susan's brother, anything was better than spending two weeks at home with his sister. Little did he realise the horror of the alternative he was given, though.

There would be no appeal.

*

Tuesdays and Thursdays at Oak House

Oak House was a single story building at the east end of the St Augustine's site in open, grassed fields used for grazing, just a few minutes' walk from Beech House. A single storey building, it was set just below the level of the surrounding ground, in an area which was later protected by Kent County Council as a 'Special Landscape Area'.

*

"Why is that man shaking Ted?"

"It's because they are pulsing 600 milliamps of current through his brain every six seconds."

"Oh, so it's a Tuesday or a Thursday then."

"It's a Tuesday."

"Why do they let us see it?"

"Because they don't care what we think, because they think everyone here is mad."

"Even me?"

"You're not, though you're here."

"Why do they do it?"

"To make people better. This advanced treatment means that they can build careers cooking the brains of these patients – men who were unlucky enough to be born with a different chemical balance in their brains, men who were already different and even abused for their differences, some who were just unlucky to have accidents."

For a young boy in an adult mental hospital, days of the week were relatively meaningless. There were more important things to worry about, being stuck in a ward with very seriously disturbed adult male patients. Nevertheless, Susan's brother always knew when it was a Tuesday or a Thursday at the hospital. And, he still asked Ted the same question twice a week.

Tuesdays and Thursdays in the Nightingale Ward 'C'.

On Tuesday and Thursday afternoons, the porters worked their way methodically along the ward, wheeling the patients one by one through to the adjacent, open, treatment area. Susan's brother could see it clearly.

Another patient, another brain. Inject a relaxant. Shave the patches, wheel him in, apply the gel, attach the electrodes, check the 'dosage' level, set the timers, switch the machine on. Push the start button. Induce a seizure.

Somewhere, probably to the west, probably in Didcot, along the railway line - Brunel's Great Western Line – another ton of coal went into the boilers, to heat the water, produce the steam, spin the turbines and push the electrons at 132,000 volts eastwards at the speed of light, on the pylons across the fields, down the cables under the streets, into the machine.

And then, through the electrodes attached to the shaven area of the skull. Through, the skin, the bone, the soft grey tissue the electrons flowed, changing who knew which synapses, which cells, in who knew what way.

Or maybe the electrons came from Dartford, it didn't really matter. Who could tell?

Every electron was the same, every brain was different.

Still, it was leading-edge medicine.

It worked.

Sometimes.

There were statistically supportable therapeutic gains, for some patients.

Sometimes it didn't work, sometimes, for some patients, so the statistics said.

Modern medicine in action.

Just as blood-letting had been modern in its time.

Lobotomies too.

Scientific progress.

Electroconvulsive therapy ('ECT') could be administered in many ways – unilateral, bifrontal, with different currents, pulse lengths, voltages and power settings. There had been many experiments, many brains treated. Many protocols had been tried and developed almost since electricity had first been 'invented' and used as a means of torture, execution even. What possessed that first person to attach electrodes to someone's skull and initiate this chain of events? It started somewhere, at a specific place and one point in time. Then its popularity grew amongst medical professionals and torturers, even executioners.

Before starting to repair the abnormal brain, before the first ECT treatment session for a particular patient, the doctor had to determine that patient's seizure threshold.

"What's a seizure threshold, Ted?"

"It's a trial and error method where they increase the stimulus – that's the electric current – to the brain, until the patient has a seizure. It's very scientific – they call it dose titration.

Then, they add fifty percent and that becomes the patient's regular dose. They record it in the patient's medical records, so they'll know next time."

"What's a seizure?"

"I think it's when the brain locks up."

"Ughh. I don't like the sound of that. And fifty percent?"

"Half. They add half as much again, just to be sure. That's medical science, precise."

Wheel that one out, still trembling and drooling from the seizure, but otherwise quiescent. Treatment successful for today. Wheel another one in.

Afternoons, Tuesdays and Thursdays in Ward 'C'.

The procedure was repeated many times over in many hospitals worldwide. Different days, perhaps, and alternative protocols for the treatment, maybe, but the brains were individual, each one unique, grown, fed and developed from that most ancient of unions between two genetic codes, stretching back to the primordial soup.

Many brains were born out of basic biological programming, the chemical drive to replicate, hurriedly, urgently, whilst alive and fertile, with no further commitment. A few were born out of love, with lifelong commitment ahead. Fewer still were born out of crime. None were yet born out of artificial unions. That was still years away in the future.

Whatever the reason was for their creation was unimportant – the brains' cells multiplied as they began to control the organism which fed and housed them.

Some brains would be considered abnormal before they had reached adult size. Unfortunately, a small percentage would be abnormal for many years before diagnosis as result of some aberrant social or criminal behaviour.

At some time in its history each brain in Ward 'C' would have been adjudged abnormal on a scale set by the mental health professionals, but also by mores of behaviour.

In the Soviet Union, people who disagreed with the State could be considered abnormal and incarcerated in a mental hospital for such corrective treatment. In such countries, politics and convenience were two additional categories against which to judge the 'normality' of a brain and the personality it realised.

In England, doctors were more enlightened. The definitions of illness and damage were narrower in extent. The treatment, though, was the same, and standards of care were higher.

Physical damage, be it accidental or criminal, illness, disease, mutation or just poor 'schooling' (in the broadest sense of a brain learning its business) were all causes of abnormality in the brains of Ward 'C'.

Thousands of measured doses every week around the world. Throw the switches, watch the dials, fill in the forms, collect the statistics, analyse the results, write the papers, attend the conferences. Each paper a step forward, another publication, another line on the CV.

Each statistic was a person with an abnormal brain, with a personality which might be changed for ever. Or not.

Scientific.

Therapeutic.

Leading edge.

This was 1957, and research was still progressing, as it does even today. The classification of mental 'problems' was still being refined; as statistical data and doctors' reports were collated (without the use of computers), 'new' syndromes and abnormal conditions were being described in the literature. Some syndromes were as yet 'undiscovered', though the evidence was buried in the data.

"Does anybody really care, Ted?"

"Yes, many of the doctors and consultants do care, in an abstract way, and some people are cured – whatever that means."

"What's abstract?"

"I think it means 'something taken out'."

"Oh - and what's a consultant?"

"Someone who knows more than a doctor and is called Mister."

"They must know a lot then - the doctors know loads. At least they don't wire me up – why's that?"

"Because you are not ill or damaged in the same way as the others are."

"But everyone tells me I can't read or write, and no one will ever want me. I'll never get anywhere in life. Isn't that why I'm here? There must be a reason."

"If you think that, why ask? It's not true, and it's not illness anyway."

"Then why am I in a hospital? Come to that, it's not really a hospital is it? It's a nuthouse! Why am I here – and don't mention that Vicar again?"

"Ask Mother."

"You keep saying that. You know she doesn't talk to me. Well, hardly at all."

"Maybe she doesn't know how to talk to you, doesn't understand boys."

"Maybe, but I'm her son. She talks to Susan, cuddles her. I never get any hugs. She's put me here."

"No, you said to her on that trip to Canterbury that you wouldn't go home if Susan was there. So, you ended up here. What else could they do?"

"It's not right, not right. I shouldn't be here with these madmen. I'll never forget this ward. And the smell, it's horrible on Tuesday and Thursday afternoons. It hangs around for ages. Ughh."

Smells lingered.

Smells reinforced memory.

A young growing brain has billions of fresh cells, the potential for trillions of synapses to lay down memories.

The oldest memories are the most tenacious.

Tuesday and Thursday in Ward 'C', afternoons.

Oak House embraced Ward 'C', at the eastern end of the site of St. Augustine's, in 1958, and staff there attempted to treat the worst of the worst patients, in societal terms - those one tier below the criminally insane or who were otherwise a danger to society. But why was a nine year old boy there, with these seriously disturbed adult males?

Why was he seeing modern mental medicine in action?

Above all, why did his middle-class, middle-England, post-war respectable mother consent to this treatment?

*

Oak House had its positive side for Susan's brother too.

"It's a complicated game."

"I'm getting the hang of it though."

"Sid's a good bloke, he makes chess interesting."

"Well it is - it's a battle, with two armies."

"I know that, but I never played before, always thought it was a stupid waste of time. And compl'cated too."

"Why, you got anything better to do then?"

"Not really. Sid helps me understand the moves, and 'strategy' he says – whatever that is. He explains things, takes time with me, shows an interest in me. Not many people do that."

"Helps you to think?"

"S'pose so, but it's not like the doctors prescribed it, and Sid's a patient here too, not a doctor, so how can he be helping me? We're just passing the time.

"Stupid boys can't play chess."

"What's that supposed to mean?"

"Whatever you think."

"What kind of answer is that?"

"Think about it, like you think about a move when you play chess."

"You're daft."

"No I'm not, I'm Ted, remember. Part of you. Anyway what's Sid in for then?"

"He told me that his wife doesn't want him. Kicked him out of the house."

"Did he try to top himself?"

Don't know, but he said he got depressed, couldn't see the point of going on."

"Didn't they give him tablets?"

"What, for his wife?"

"No you berk, for his being depressed an' that."

"Don't know. He's here, whatever. I think the chess helps him too."

"Has he got any kids?"

"A boy an' a girl I heard. It must hurt him, being kicked out, being here, not seeing them."

"What do you mean by hurt?"

"You know, missing them, like you miss your mouse."

"Sort of inside, like?"

"Yeh."

"Didn't think of it like that."

"Maybe you are a substitute and he teaches you what he can't teach his son?"

"Like chess you mean?"

"Yeh, and bar billiards too."

"Who'll teach his son chess and bar billiards then if he can't see them?"

"Dunno."

"Sad."

"Yeh, sad. But at least he's teaching you. Father would probably be teaching you if he hadn't died."

"Yeh, if he hadn't died I wouldn't be in here either."

"Maybe. But Sid's children would still be without *their* Dad."

Sid Coombes was to become a family friend. Although he was a patient at Oak House, his interest in Susan's brother helped the ten year old boy, and perhaps helped Sid himself.

The staff cottages were at the south western end of the site, bordering Chartham Downs Road, and sheltered from the north wind by a deep copse of trees. They were not full family homes, suitable only a maximum of two people. Of course, no staff would want to raise a family on this site, and no normal child going to school would want to admit living in the grounds of a mental hospital.

"Bill seemed pleased to see me."

"Yes, just married and they don't have much money – they couldn't even go on honeymoon."

"Not sure I'd fancy a honeymoon painting a cottage."

"Yes, but he's got his new wife there with him, every night."

"I wonder what it's like?"

"What, painting a cottage?"

"No, you berk. Sleeping with a woman, you know messing around."

"Dunno. I wonder if she farts."

"Probably. No escape though if you're under the same blankets."

"Anyway, it was nice of him to take me to the fair. Rides, toffee apple – he paid for the lot. Fantastic! What was best though was the ride on his motorbike."

"What was it?"

"AJS 350 single. I'll never forget it."

"Makes a hell of a noise though."

"Yeh, but what a great feeling. Power throbbing between the legs. Brmm, brmm"

"That's enough. Stop it. Go to sleep."

"OK."

*

"That was a nice walk. Walks get me away from people."

"All the walks round here are nice."

"Yes, it was nice to meet someone who seems to care about me."

"Are you meeting Dennis again?"

"I hope so – he seems to be there every time I go that way."

"Do you believe what he says about taking you to South Africa?"

"Yes, I'm going to start planning what I'll need to take. I'm going to smoke less and save some of the ciggie money."

"Do you like what he asks you to do to him?"

"I know he's as bent as a nine-bob note, but I don't think about it. He cares for me, he's taking me with him to South Africa. Away from here. I will have a new life."

"Why South Africa?"

"I don't know, but he seems to know a lot about it. Says we'll have a maid and all, to look after me."

"Blimey, that'll be brilliant!"

"Yeh, can't wait."

"How are you going to get there?"

"Dunno – maybe a ship or a plane – he hasn't told me."

"A ship! Cor, you might get seasick!"

"What's that?"

"Dunno really, I heard that people get sick on ships that's all."

"Well, it'll be worth it, for a maid. I'd prefer a plane though. Quicker too."

"What colour do you reckon she'll be?"

"What, the ship or the maid?"

"The maid you berk!"

"Oh. Dunno, Dennis'll know. They're all black out there anyway aren't they. Zulus an' that. Spears and stuff."

"Don't be daft!"

"I'll ask Dennis."
Dennis was one of the adult patients at Oak House.

*

"Have you got everything?"
"I think so."
"How will we get to South Africa?"
"Dennis knows how. He's got it all planned. I'd better go."

*

After everyone thought he had gone to bed – and he thought everyone was asleep - Susan's brother put a pillow under his bedclothes and slipped out of Oak House. Every stair tread seemed to creak, every door hinge squealed – at least, that's how it seemed to him. He couldn't really hear much beyond the sound of his blood pumping in his ears as his heart beat quickly, and the noises he heard disturbed no-one, though his imagination amplified them. He was very nervous, as he tip-toed downstairs and his normal awkwardness was made worse by the tension in his limbs – he felt like a puppet as he tried to creep through the entrance hall and his legs trembled. Then, he eased the front door open and moved around the outside of the building.

It was just getting dark as he headed round the back, trying to keep in the shadows, through the gate and down the path towards Beech Toll where there had been a toll gate, many years ago. He crossed the road and opened the gate into the field. Keeping to the hedge, he could just see the low profile of Oak House through the trees to the north, behind him. He sat down and waited at the agreed meeting place, under the broad oak at the edge of Rabbit Wood gazing south with a magnificent aspect over the Downs in the Spring twilight.

"He's late."
"Maybe I got the time wrong."
"How long are you going to wait?"
"'Till he comes."
"Supposing he doesn't?"
"He will."

"But what if he doesn't?"

"I don't know. Stop nagging me – I'm nervous enough as it is. Going on a ship to a new country, a new life. I'm scared stiff."

The twilight was bright behind him, to the northwest, as Susan's brother sat under the tree, the tree where he had first met Dennis and where he'd been shown affection, and other things. He didn't think of home, he didn't think of Mother, and he certainly didn't think of Susan. The dusk settled in slowly – it was a clear night and at this time of the year, close to midsummer's day, it would not get really dark at all.

He started as he heard some rustling in the undergrowth, and watched a fox walk out boldly onto the path. It passed him less than six feet away, not stopping, and ignoring him completely.

"Shit, that scared me! I thought it was Dennis!"

"I don't reckon he's coming."

"He'll come."

"Are you sure?"

"No I'm not. Grown-ups always let me down, don't they? Just like those men in the butcher's shop."

"Yeh. Maybe he will come. But how would you get money in South Africa?"

"Dennis said he's get a job and look after me."

"Well, he'd better bloody hurry up."

"Shut up, I'm getting cold."

"It's nerves, that what it is."

"Maybe."

"He makes me laugh."

"I know."

"Where is he then? Why hasn't he come? Do they lock them in at night?"

"Don't know. Maybe he's had an accident, or some other problem. Gosh – maybe he got caught leaving!"

"They'll know about me bunking off then. He'd never split on me though."

A barn owl hooted nearby and he jumped again as another returned the call from a tree on the other side of the field.

"That's enough, I'm not staying out here all night. Too many wild animals."

"They're only owls and foxes and things, nothing dangerous."

"I'm not taking the chance, there's still just enough light for me to find my way back. I'm off."

Slowly, Susan's brother picked his way along the path to the gate.

"It's late and everyone will be asleep. If I get back soon, they will not think I've run away. I'll have to sneak in carefully – I just hope I can find an open window."

"Why don't you go in the way you came out?"

"Don't be daft, I didn't leave it on the latch, I was going to Africa."

"That's rich that is."

"What?"

"You climbing in through the window."

"Why?"

"Well, you ended up here because you tried to climb out of that window at Epping House."

"Yeh, well things are different now."

"How come?"

"Dunno, just different."

"You've given up thinking of suicide then?"

"No, but, well, but – oh stop asking stupid questions!"

"Not stupid!"

"Yes it is!"

"No. Maybe it's them tablets?"

"P'raps. I don't know. Shut up or we'll wake them up."

"Hear us! Are you nuts? I'm in your head."

"Oh, right. Well, leave me alone – I've got to be very quiet while I get back upstairs to the dorm, otherwise I'll wake somebody and there'll be all hell raised."

Susan's brother continued his walks after that day, but never saw Dennis again.

"I reckon Dennis never intended to take me anywhere. He just wanted to fiddle around. I never did though, and I never will."

"You said he was nice, though."

"Yeh, he was nice, but he lied to me. Why do all grown-ups have to lie all the time."

"Not all of them do. Sid Coombes doesn't."

"S'pose so."

"Why do some of the men want to fiddle around? I keep well away from them?"

"Dunno. Maybe it's because there are no girls here?"

"Could be."

"Don't know when I'll have my first kiss though."

"It'll happen. Bound to."

"What if she smokes? Would you kiss her then?"

"Yeh, s'pose so, but at least she'd be wearing scent."

"Maybe, but she wouldn't drink it would she? Her mouth would still taste of ciggies."

"Well yours does."

"Don't be stupid, of course it does, it's mine!"

"Well, they keep it closed when they kiss, like in the films."

"Best way I reckon, though it's not what the other boys say – I'm not sure I fancy tongues. French kissing the boys call it. Ughh."

"Shh, I think someone's coming!"

Susan's brother heard the lavatory flush as he slipped back into bed, and then a door closed at the end of the corridor. His heart was still racing, and he fought with thoughts of disappointment and betrayal. Eventually, he fell asleep dreaming of owls and foxes, in a place his dream told him was South Africa though he had never seen a picture or held any conscious image of the country.

*

Back to Beech House

After the short but intensive holiday experience at Oak House, Beech House re-opened and Susan's brother returned, but with little real relief at the prospect. It was, though, infinitely better than being at home with Susan.

The mornings at Beech House were taken up by school. There was no formal teaching – the boys were left to self-study, mainly reading.

"I've had enough, Ted. I wish I had front teeth."

"They're bound to grow."

"Keith is the worst."

"Yes, I hate him, I hate them all."

"Be patient, your eye will improve and your teeth will grow."

"There's no sign of my teeth. I am just ugly. I can't even play football properly."

"You try."

*

"Did I do all right?"

"You fixed him good."

"Maybe I went too far."

"He needed a good lesson - you stood up for yourself and gave him a hiding."

"At least Keith knows that I can fight, and I can hurt him."

"Yes, a bloody nose, and his teeth too."

"That makes up for all the times he laughed at my gap."

"He's got one of his own now."

"I still don't like fighting."

"It's just as well there were no teachers around."

"I hope he won't grass on me."

"I doubt it – he'll probably say he fell downstairs or banged into a door."

"Serves him right."

"Yeh, he had it coming. Nick taught you well."

As the boys fell asleep, there was a different mood in the dormitory, and a change of focus. Now that Susan's brother had beaten Keith, another boy, Stephen Cartwright, who was the next weakest in line, became the target of the bullying. Keith was nursing a bloody nose and an embarrassing gap where there should have been front teeth - things would not be the same again since Susan's brother had, at last, stood up for himself. For Cartwright the nightmare was just beginning.

It was one small step, but a hugely important confidence-building step for a small and introverted boy. He had learned the hard way to stand up to bullies, without any guidance from a father.

*

More Change at Home

In 1958, whilst Susan's brother was in Beech House, Valerie had moved home, to South Park Gardens.

Geoff Gower, who used to play golf with Roy, had suggested to Valerie that she buy one of the new chalet bungalows being built in South Park Gardens, Berkhamsted. The move was completed in 1958, selling Dell Field Close for £50 more than the purchase price (£3,500) of the new, much bigger, property.

This was a time of great expansion, as new dormitory towns were constructed all around London. Harold Macmillan's words seemed to be bearing fruit and after the shock of the war, there were new ideas emerging about society and urban planning, which had triggered the New Towns act of 1946. Stevenage, Letchworth, Welwyn Garden City (with Hatfield) and Borehamwood were nearby Hertfordshire's early contribution.

At the time of Valerie's move to South Park Gardens, only one side of the road had been built. When all the houses had been built, the builders started on the other side.

*

Secondary School Level

At Easter in 1959, Susan's brother left Beech House. He had progressed at Beech House in some ways, but had not been happy there – happiness was a state of mind alien to him. His mother had visited him half a dozen times, and his sister once, under protest, on that dreadful day that he had been assigned to Oak House for the holidays.

On his last day at Beech House, he caught the late morning train from Canterbury to London. He carried all his worldly possessions in a small case, the most important items – a radio and some magazines underneath a few clothes and a toothbrush. Mickey had long gone and had not been replaced - his cage had been taken away in the rubbish lorry. Susan's brother knew that there would be little at home that he would recognise as his. Recollections are of a sunny day as the train wound through the blossoming orchards of Kent towards London. Anyone in the carriage looking at him would have seen a ten year-old boy who was clearly unhappy and burdened.

He was in no hurry to get to Berkhamsted and broke the journey at Bromley where he bought a soft drink at the station café. As he sat on a station bench he reflected on the day.

"I never thought I'd ever get out of Beech House. I thought I'd be stuck in a special school for ever. Now here I am on my own on a railway station, and I've just bought myself a bottle of pop. I feel free, but it's not going to last is it? It feels really weird. I'm scared."

"Well, you are growing up - they had to send you somewhere. You're too old to stay there any longer. You've got to go out into the world."

"I'm severely disturbed, that's what they say. I'm surprised they've let me out."

"You are getting better, not talking about suicide."

"Maybe. But where will I go next? And now, today, I've got to go home and spend Easter with Susan. It's a nightmare starting all over again."

"Maybe Mum knows what your next school will be and she'll tell you when you get home."

"I hope so. She must know – the holiday is only two weeks long. At least Susan will be going back to her school then, but it's the two weeks I'm dreading. Not only that, everything is new. They even moved house without telling me."

"Just be patient for a couple of weeks."

"That's easy to say, but you know Susan, you know what she will say, how she will treat me – she's ashamed of me. It's a nightmare."

He hadn't imagined being free from special schools and hospitals ever again, and he hadn't imagined that he would ever go home again. Now, he was dreading the time to be spent at home before he went to wherever would be next – the not knowing was almost as bad as the prospect of two weeks at home with his sister. Intellectually, he was constrained by the special school system and couldn't think his way out of it; emotionally he was drained by the prospect of being at home with Susan again.

Mother met him at Victoria Station and they had lunch at a station café after emerging from the Tube at Euston to await their train.

Over lunch he discovered that the educational psychologists had recommended that his secondary schooling should be at Boxmoor House, the senior school for Epping House where he had failed to end his life. Normal boys would have gone to Apsley Grammar, or Ashlyns Secondary Modern School. Not so Susan's brother – he was still trapped in the special school system as a boarder. As far as he was concerned, boarding anywhere was infinitely better than living at home, whatever the school.

Beyond the discussion of his next school – and that was very one-sided, Mother was not able to engage with the lad – the communication gap was as big as ever and attempts at conversation were strained. After all, there was little to talk about – there was no shared family life, and the lonely boy had no interest in Susan's exploits and he was in some trepidation about the new house. The forty minute ride on the Berkhamsted train passed in silence, the final leg of the journey to a home he had never seen, a bedroom he had never slept in, the two cats, and his sister.

During his year at Beech house, there had been some sort of stability, a pattern to his unhappy life but now all that was changing. Apart from a short Christmas visit, he had been away for a year and there was little in common in their lives.

The afternoon spring sunshine was warm as they strolled from the station, along a route that he was not familiar with, down a new road, into a new estate, with unknown neighbours, into an uncertain future. They walked up past the front lawn and Mother opened the door with her key. Susan heard the latch and appeared in the hallway.

She smiled and said hello to her mother as she hugged her, and then turned to her brother. A young boy arriving at a new home after a year away would normally expect some interest, excitement, perhaps, from a loving, welcoming sister – perhaps even:

"Come on, I'll show you your new bedroom!"

It was not to be.

The look on her face was one of great disappointment and her words were harsh and wounding, devoid of concern or love.

He was an interloper on her territory. And the message she gave was uncompromising:

"Well, now that you are home, I suppose I shall have to tell all the neighbours that you are mentally ill. My friends too."

She turned, without another word and went directly upstairs to her bedroom.

Her brother had not expected anything different. Indeed, such an attitude was why he hadn't wanted to go home for the summer holidays, and why he had endured the experience in Oak House.

No, nothing had changed at home, except the home itself. 'Home' as a concept meant nothing to him. He had been upset when he had heard that Mother was moving from Dell Field Close, so perhaps there was some emotional link or bond to that house where he had last seen his father.

Number 14 South Park Gardens had been a complete mystery to him – he had not even seen any photographs. Unlike boys in other families moving home, he had not shared in the excitement of the buying process, in the packing and preparing, in the moving or in the first night at the new residence. He felt no feeling of 'ownership' or excitement in the way that any typical child would in a new home. There was no desire to explore, all that lay ahead was a dreaded holiday with Susan.

His few possessions had been moved for him, his wardrobe and chest of drawers packed, moved and unpacked. Any clothes would no longer fit him, though his train set and Lancaster bomber had survived the journey. It was just another place, another bed – one of many in which he'd slept in over the last few years.

Mother and the cats had settled in, and Susan had her bedful of soft cuddly toys, and a normal life.

Though he probably didn't realise it at the time, he was marginally more resilient, marginally stronger emotionally, better able to cope with other people and new situations. After all, he'd coped with Keith, and climbed a rung up the ladder out of the pit. There were many more rungs before he could hope to reach his sister's level, but that was not something he considered, or aspired to.

So, another first night spent in another bed – that was all it seemed to be to him.

It still hurt him that he was a disappointment to Susan. He was clearly a brother she would rather not have. After all, he couldn't give her money or introduce her to nice boys. He didn't know what he could do to make her happy.

It hurt him that his mother had moved from Dell Field Close, and that first night he fell asleep looking forward to leaving again. He didn't feel part of a family, he just felt like a stranger in a strange house.

*

"I'm fed up. Mum's moved here without telling me. Why did she have to leave Dell Field Close?"

"Dunno."

"All these new people."

"Yes, well some of them are really nice."

"Yeh, but now there are more people to think I'm at a special school. Everyone knows what that means. Not only that, the boys at Boxmoor will be the same ones who were at Epping House. It's just the same nightmare in another place."

"Boxmoor is not a Borstal. You're not a criminal, you've just been ill. It'll get better."

*

Along with move of house, Mother had also moved from her job at Kilfillan School and was working for Television Audience Measurement (TAM) which was an essential component in the television advertising world. A TAM box had been installed next to the Bush 14" black and white television set at South Park Gardens, although the Robinson household was far from typical in audience measurement terms.

In the late summer of 1958, Susan's brother was at home and new neighbours were moving in, week by week.

The Tolhursts were one of the first families to move in across the road, about six months after Susan's brother left Beech House.

Geoff Gower was a neighbour, and Susan's brother became friendly with the Gower boys, Richard and Peter. The building site – North Park Gardens – was exciting for the young boys. At about 4.30 pm when the builders had left for the day, the boys would enter the site through a gap in the fence, and explore. In those far off days there was little in the way of formal Health and Safety regulations, and builders had a relatively high accident rate.

*

The Fonz

In September 2011, it was announced that Henry Winkler, a US citizen aged 65 years old, was being awarded an Honorary OBE, for his work on raising awareness of dyslexia. Winkler had made his name as 'The Fonz' – an ultra-cool youth in a US sitcom called 'Happy Days' about the carefree days of a group of US teenagers living in the American Dream. The sitcom and its theme tune had resonated with the youth of the time, way back in the 1970s, and was a massive hit. Production ceased only when Winkler was too old to convincingly portray a teenager. Winkler, though, had a learning difficulty, something which none of his hundreds of thousands of teenage fans knew about, though many of them shared.

Winkler was dyslexic.

The condition Dyslexia (often known as word blindness) has several different symptoms, any or all which may present in a person. These include 'jumping words' when reading, difficulty in focusing the eyes quickly when scanning a sentence, poor balance, clumsiness – particularly poor hand/eye coordination, distorted perception.

Simple tasks such as tying shoelaces can be very difficult. Confusion between right and left, and difficulty telling the time on a clock with hands are all quite common symptoms which can make daily life very challenging.

Henry Winkler's OBE was awarded for his having written seventeen children's books and his tireless visiting of British schools to explain his condition. He had suffered in school form being a slow learner, and as an actor had struggled to read scripts. But people with a disability compensate in other ways, and The Fonz was no exception. It was not until he was 31 years old that his dyslexia ('word blindness') was diagnosed.

The award of an OBE is a great honour, particularly when the recipient is not a UK citizen.

Boxmoor House Special School

Boxmoor House Special School is close to the village of Boxmoor, near Hemel Hempstead. The village itself, near the River Bulbourne, dates back many centuries – millennia even - and is a district of Dacorum. This is a clue as to its long history. A Roman villa (English Heritage Monument No.359304) was discovered in the grounds of Boxmoor House in 1851, and subsequently re-excavated in 1966 and 1969 when Boxmoor House School was being extended.

The village itself enjoys some notoriety, as the site of the last legal execution where the victim was buried at the scene of the crime. Robert Snooks, a highwayman, robbed a post boy on the turnpike near Boxmoor Meadows, and was hung and buried near the spot in 1802. The location of his remains is marked today by two stones.

In 1958, Boxmoor House was the senior-school equivalent of Epping House, the senior school for the 'malads' as the maladjusted boys were known. Many of the boys there had been fellow-pupils of Susan's brother at Epping House, so going to Boxmoor was in some ways, for him, taking a step back in time and reviving painful memories. Not all patients were 'malads' – there were some who boarded because of difficult home circumstances, ranging from physical neglect to problems with parents, step-parents and 'lodgers'. Other boys had criminal records which were not serious enough to warrant being in an approved school or a borstal.

The boys slept in dormitories, in three separate groups: Ages 11-12, 12-14 and 14+. At the age of 15, they would move out to their own accommodation, and hopefully started work full time, with maybe night school for the cleverer ones. That was what the education policies were geared towards. Unfortunately, the reality usually fell short of those laudable aspirations.

The headmaster was R. A. Carrington, known to one and all as 'The Boss". He was a tolerant, perceptive and able Head who was respected by staff and boys alike. The Boss would prove to be just the right Head at just the right time for Susan's brother, who started as a full-time boarder in Boxmoor in September 1958.

It would be, for him, a key school in his future. In the meantime, he had a lot of baggage and the first year was difficult as he struggled to get used to 'school routine' again; his emotional state, though, continued to improve. Occasionally though, unhappy memories came back to haunt him.

*

"What are you doing?"

"Writing a letter."

"It looks nasty."

"It is. That bastard Mel Perkins should have let me jump. I fucking hate him for stopping me."

"Stop swearing – Father would be cross with you."

"Father's not here, he's dead, remember?"

"You shouldn't get at Mel. He couldn't let you jump – it was his job to stop you. Not only that, he was concerned for you."

"Concerned? No chance. No-one cares for me."

"Yes they do. What about Mr. Vernon, Mr. Draper, Mr. Turl or Sid Coombes. Remember the Matron at the North Mid? She was lovely. Lots of them care."

"It's just their job, they do it for pay. And Sid was just a patient. And don't forget Mr. Case and taking our clothes off. Head Case he was! They are not all good."

"Yeh, OK. But you can't send that letter."

"I will."

"Then don't use such nasty words. You shouldn't be writing things like that in a letter. It's not right."

"I don't care. That's what I feel."

"He will recognise the handwriting on the envelope."

"No he won't. John is going to write the address for me."

"That's sly."

"Yes. I hate the bastard and I want him to know it."

*

The regime at Boxmoor was fairly relaxed, but there were also some distinctly unusual aspects. Susan's brother wondered why the boys' shower time was supervised by the teachers' wives, one of whom is remembered even today for being attractive, with bright red lipstick and low cut blouses.

Even in the youngest age group, some of the boys had reached puberty. One boy in particular, Scargill, always hid from whichever lady was in the changing room supervising showers, because of his very obvious engorgement.

"I don't understand it. Why do the teachers' wives have to supervise the showers?"

"It is weird. Maybe they think we'll get up to something."

"Well, that stuff happens anyway, showers or no showers."

"Yeh, you're right. Having women around doesn't bother me, but Scargill seems to have a big problem with it, hiding like that."

"Yeh, see what you mean about a big problem."

"Wolfey's wife seems to dress up 'specially for it too."

"Strange, isn't it?"

"Yeh. 'Least I don't have to run and hide myself."

"Don't know why we need to be supervised anyway."

"Me neither."

"Still it's not like Epping House – at least I don't have to run around without clothes on."

"I don't want to think about that."

"No, but I can understand how Scargill feels."

What were the reasons for this? We can only speculate – were the male staff absent so that any dubious behaviour with the boys could be avoided? Or, perhaps, it was quite the reverse, and the boys were to be stimulated, as Scargill evidently was? Most boys' schools will have male teachers in the changing rooms after sports, even today.

*

After six months in Boxmoor, he was at home during the holiday when he met the new neighbours.

"You like the Tolhursts - we may see Mrs. Tolhurst now, and she may ask us in for tea."

"Why can't everyone be like the Tolhursts?"

"Because there is good and evil in the world. We learn that in church on Sundays."

"And I see it every day, I feel it every day, this evil. It hurts me, upsets me. Why do we go to church Ted?"

"To talk to God."

"We talk to God in school at assembly, but he never answers back. He doesn't exist."

"There are a lot of people for him to talk to."

"He never talks to anyone – none of the other boys say he talks to them. Why?"

"He does talk to them and to you, maybe you can't hear him."

"There's no point in life."

"Don't start that again, you must keep trying."

"Why?"

"Because God loves us and we should love God."

"God doesn't exist, why do you keep on about him?"

"Because everyone says he is there for us, to help us, to love us."

"What's love?"

"You keep asking that. The answer's still the same."

"OK, but what's the point in life?"

"Ask the Tolhursts – maybe Bob knows."

"Yes, he knows a lot. And they even call me by my name."

"They see you differently to the way that Mother and Susan do. They care about you."

"I don't know how much longer I can stand this. Susan keeps telling me that no-one will ever want me and that I'll never get anywhere in life. At least she's stopped saying that I'm fat and clumsy. Are there other Tolhursts in the world Ted?"

"I don't know."

"I always look forward to Tuesday nights."

"Yeh, they're brilliant."

"Tea and TV with them. Is that what normal families are like?

"'Prob'ly."

"Maybe we'd have been like that if Father was alive, and I wouldn't have to go to these stupid schools."

"Could be, but you'll never know."

"Three daughters, and they're all nice. Why can't Susan be like them?"

"Good question, but how should I know the answer? Briony's your age – you might have a chance with her."

"Yeh. Vivienne's nice too. Shame about that patch on her specs covering her left eye."

"It's only till her eye strengthens. You had your teeth to worry about. Nobody's perfect. Look at Susan – she looks pretty and she's clever, but she's not a nice person, at least not to me."

"I suppose you're right. And even Jennifer is nice, though she's only a toddler. She's cute."

"Yeh. It must be nice to have a little sister like that."

"I really like Briony, though."

"And she's the same age."

"Yeh."

"Do you fancy her then?"

"Dunno, never really thought about it. I think she's probably more like the sister I wish I had."

*

Other neighbours in South Park Gardens included the Ayres family, the Balchins and the Tebbits.

Gerry Ayres was a manager at Dickersons, a local printing firm.

Norman Tebbit (now Lord Tebbit) was an airline pilot with BOAC (having joined them in 1953 from the RAF) and also an official with the British Airline Pilots' Association.

*

His first year at Boxmoor was difficult, and the taunting about his speech continued. Just as we cannot choose our families, we cannot, as children, choose our environment. The learning of speech is osmotic and automatic; accent and pronunciation are absorbed from the family first, and adjusted in concert with one's peers as schooling begins and progresses. Susan's brother was not given elocution lessons, but his family's speech was middle class, his pronunciation generally correct and reflective of that background.

At Boxmoor, as had been the case at Epping House and Beech House, the bulk of the patients were drawn from family backgrounds where the manner of speech was, for want of a better phrase, less cultured.

This was clearly something that his sister would not have criticised him for, but was glaringly obvious in the special schools.

Gradually, Susan's brother lost some of the 'cultured tone' of his accent, and his speech started to reflect that of his peer group.

*

Mother's attitude had improved since Susan's brother had been in Beech House and as he was maturing and stabilising at Boxmoor House. Her treatment of him was better, but still well below the way that he perceived she treated Susan.

"Mum's nicer to me, but Susan's got worse. First she told her friends I was mentally ill when I got home from Beech House. Now she only says that to me."

"You're not mentally ill."

"No, now she just keeps on about God having punished her with a brother like me. I don't want her to tell anyone that, especially Briony."

"She shouldn't say things like that."

"No, and there's no God to punish her anyway. It doesn't matter. I hate going home when she's there."

*

When he was 11, and at home for the summer holidays, his mother arranged a holiday for him. She put him on a train to London and at Euston he was met by an adult supervisor; they went with a group of other children on a week's camping holiday, out in fields near Heathrow. Although the A4 was busy, the area was in those days relatively undeveloped, with none of the motorway infrastructure, business parks and multiple airport terminals that we see today. The group was mixed, and Susan's brother started to make friends with the opposite sex.

"Susan Wallingford did say she'd write."

"I know, but I didn't think she would. I never get letters at school."

"The Boss's face was a picture. I can see him holding that envelope and feeling it with fingers and hear him now:

'I've had an interesting letter for Robinson, and to me it feels suspiciously as though it contains a cigarette.' At least he was smiling as he said it."

"Yeh, but I was embarrassed."

"Well, he didn't open it and read it, so that's ok. What did she say anyway?"

"Nothing."

"Nothing? Just a cigarette? You're having me on!"

"Mind your own business then."

*

"Do you think that Mother cares for me?"

"Yeh, 'course she does, why do you keep asking?"

"Well, maybe things are changing. Since I left Beech House, I think she's been more – ermm – well – more like a mother I suppose, though I don't really know what that means. Maybe like Mrs. Tolhurst, or like Tim's mum used to be."

"Tim who?"

"Y'know, where they didn't have enough plates, down off Swingate Lane. Used to go there for tea. No carpets either, but at least he had a blue blazer, a proper blazer for school, not a stupid green girl's blazer like me."

"Oh, that Tim, with the two sisters."

"Yes. Haven't seen him for ages. He stopped coming to school."

"Yeh, wonder what happened to him? Anyway, Mother seems to ask more questions, talk to you a bit more."

"She still treats Susan so much better than me – the light shines out of Susan's..."

"Stop there! Susan's a girl. Mother's a woman. Women are different. You know that."

"Yeh, I remember. Nurse Hill's. Different all right."

"They think different to us boys."

"Susan always got pocket money. Mother never gives me any."

"Yeh, she could do, that's not fair."

"And what was all that fuss about potatoes that Susan was rambling on about?"

"Yes, she was really angry, raving mad, couldn't stop babbling about it, wasn't she. You know her, when she gets going she's talking twenty to the dozen. She was on her high horse all right, just because the school cookery teacher told her how to peel the spuds so her husband wouldn't tick her off - peeling the skins too thick – wasting potato. 'Husbands don't like that', the teacher said, according to her. What a laugh! She's off her head."

"Who – Susan or the teacher?"

"Both of them, must be."

"Peeling the spuds wrong! She's crackers. I don't care about the skins, all I want is a pile of mash. And bangers. What man would go on about the potato peelings? Must be some strange blokes around."

"You know that anyway."

"Yeh, but I can't believe her sometimes. Did you hear her?

'I want to marry a man of property who I can help with his estate, manage his house and land. I don't want a man to like me because I peel potatoes eco – eco–manicly.'

"With thin peelings."

"Yeh, that's it, but she knows the proper words. Thin peelings. 'Manage his estate'. Huh. Really poncy. Who cares about potato peelings? Most people feed them to the chickens anyway. Bob puts them on his compost heap."

"Susan's got some big ideas, wanting to be rich an' all, marry a man with a fancy car and a country house. Do you think men like that worry about potato peelings? Maybe she's right."

"Thinks she's Lady Muck she does."

"Who's Lady Muck?"

"Dunno - I heard her name somewhere, but if she's anything like Susan I'm sorry for Mr. Muck."

Birthdays came and went, they were not celebrated in school and Susan's brother received no birthday cards – they were kept at home and given to him on his next home visit.

Some other boys received cards at school.

In other respects too, the school was isolated. The boys never visited Boxmoor village itself, and had little contact with the residents. They walked to church on Sunday mornings, but this didn't require walking through the village.

*

In 1959, Susan became a Christian. It was not a matter of quiet visits to church on Sundays for her. It was much more than that, leaning towards evangelicalism.

The deep-seated, oft-repeated statement that her brother had had burned into his brain now changed.

"I don't know why God is punishing me so. All I ever wanted was a good-looking brother who had a decent job, who could give me money and introduce me to nice boys; and look what I've got!"

*

1959 was an important year, as Susan's brother began to find his feet in Boxmoor House. He was now almost twelve years old, but although Mother's disposition towards him had improved somewhat, there was still a considerable emotional distance between them. Communication was little, if any, easier than it had ever been. Indeed, he could communicate well on a day-to-day basis with the neighbours in South Park Gardens, and looked forward to seeing the Tolhurst family in particular.

Christmases are not remembered at all, not when Father was alive and not until 1959. It is unusual that a child should have no memories of Christmas before the age of twelve. Of course, the whole story of Father Christmas has little basis in truth, and Susan's brother had no trust in the words of adults. Perhaps for other children, it is the belief in Father Christmas that lays down strong childhood memories of the holiday. From 1959 onward, the recollections are of Granny and Aunty Muriel coming to stay at

South Park Gardens; at Easter and Bank Holidays, the Robinson's took the train to deParis Avenue in Bedford.

In 1959, other things were changing too, and the Western world was on the verge of a cultural revolution. New musical styles were developing rapidly, with rock and skiffle and the first dawnings of pop culture. This was helped in no small way by access to transistor radios, cheap record players and widespread availability of records. Attitudes were changing as the baby boomers started to mature and question the very nature of society and challenge the norms of the day.

*

"Who were they?"

"I think they're called The Drifters."

"What'd they come here for then? Why waste half an hour setting up all their gear on the tennis court, play a few songs and then bugger off again?"

"Re-ursal someone called it. Practicing, like."

"'ardly worth it."

"Yeh well they thought it was."

"Who fixed it up then?"

"Mr. Carrington I s'pose."

"I've never seen the tennis court used for anything before, other than our PE."

"Did you see that bloke with the big glasses?"

"Yeh, someone said his name was Hank."

"Is he American then?"

"Don't think so, but he's got a funny accent – not American."

"They can't be the same Drifters what Jimmy Saville plays on 'Teen and Twenty Club' on Radio Luxembourg, can they?"

"No, they sound different – those Americans sing with high voices. This lot use a lot of guitar sound, not so much singing. Fenders I think they call them guitars. Strato something. No singing at all with some of the songs."

"How can you have a song without singing?"

"Stop picking on me! You ask some daft questions."

"It's not daft. A song has words. What's a song without words?"

"Music."

"Yeh, guess you're right. Anyway, it's confusing having two groups with the same name."

"Yeh, s'pose so. At least the music's different."

"Yeh. Did you see those amps though?"

"Yeh, Vox AC30s."

"I bet those cost a few bob."

"Top end stuff all right. Dunno what valves they use. 807's?"

"Maybe. Doubt it. '807's are for higher frequencies, not audio stuff."

"Ok, ok don't get too techie-wot's it on me. Why don't you learn to play a guitar and join a group?"

"Me? Play a guitar? Are you mad? I can't even catch a football."

"Ok, but you can solder circuit boards."

"That's different, I don't have to move an' stuff."

"Yeh, maybe so. They sound good anyway."

"Yeh. Maybe they'll become famous. They're not bad."

"Well, they're not on Radio Luxembourg yet."

*

You've Never Had It So Good

Susan's brother was getting to know the neighbours during his visits home. They seemed to treat him more or less as a normal lad.

In particular, he developed a friendship with the Tolhursts, and with Bob especially. Bob, the head of the household, treated the lonely boy almost as a surrogate son. The Tolhursts had three daughters, so Susan's brother had no rivals within the family. He enjoyed their company, and got on well with the Tolhurst sisters.

There are memories of sunny evenings after school, when Bob had come home from work and was digging in his vegetable patch. Chatting together in the garden over cups of tea brought out by Ruth, Bob's wife, as the dying breed of steam trains ran past the end of the garden.

Bob's brain was keen – he was observant and well educated. Subjects ranged from economics, including the trade balance and interest rates, inflation and the Sterling exchange rate. Susan's brother took it all in.

Some evenings would be spent with Bob watching current affairs programs on the television.

*

"Aren't you afraid you'll slip and fall off?"

"Don't think about it."

"Why doesn't he do it himself?"

"Search me. At least it gives me something to do on weekends."

"Huh, half the day's gone before he even gets out of bed, and then he asks you to nip to the grocer's for bread and milk. Your own money too. Cheeky sod."

"Yeh he's a lazy sod all right."

"You'd think that Edna would get him up and out in the mornings. It's no way to run an electronics business. He should have a sign – "North West Electronics – Every Day's a Half Day.""

"You're right, he is lazy, but she's got the twins and Sally to look after. Keith does bugger all in the house."

"Yeh, and hardly anything in the shop either. Don't know how he makes any money."

"He doesn't pay me for a start, just odd radio spares 'n stuff."

"They're all a bit strange if you ask me. And that Sally!"

"Yeh, I'm keeping well away. It's not natural for an eight years old girl to behave like that. Don't know where she gets the ideas from."

"Too right. Keith gets some good contracts though."

"Yeh, dunno how he does it. That last one was a joke though – FBI – 'Finlays Bureau of Investigation.'"

"Yeh, good one innit 'I fitted the aerials for the FBI'. In London."

Susan's brother was gaining in confidence and found odd jobs helping the likes of Keith at North West Electronics from time to time. Other boys would have been playing football, but he was furthering his interest in radio and television technology.

*

Significant Harm

In the Children Act 1989, the term 'significant harm' replaces the terms 'child abuse' and 'neglect'. Significant harm is defined as ill-treatment or the impairment of the child's health (mental or physical) or development (physical, intellectual, emotional, social or behavioural) attributable to a lack of adequate parental care or control: section 31.

Boxmoor School –1960 Onwards

Peter B was the head boy at Boxmoor when Susan's brother arrived in 1959, an honour which he held until he left a couple of years later. He was two or three years older than Susan's brother and became a best friend. Susan's brother and Peter B would later marry two sisters.

Peter was an intelligent and well–liked boarder, at Boxmoor because of parental difficulties at home. He attended Apsley Grammar School during the day.

The time at Boxmoor was a period when Susan's brother began to catch up, learning how to enjoy life, forming strong friendships with Peter B and Terry W, and getting on well with the staff.

The headmaster of Apsley Grammar was V J Wrigley (Valentine). His wife was French and reputedly had fought in the Resistance during the war, so she was a tough and resilient woman. Mr. and Mrs. Wrigley's daughter, Diana attended Berkhamsted Girls' School, and was one of Susan's best friends there. Later, for a short time, Susan's brother was Diana's boyfriend.

*

Fellow patients were either disturbed or having problems at home, and one boy, Parsons was said to be seriously disturbed. He was smart though, in a barrow–boy way.

The staff members were perceptive and used to dealing with difficult boys – all were treated individually with a high staff/boarder ratio. Individual aptitudes were recognised, praised and encouraged.

One of the teachers was a Mr. Wolfe. He and his wife lived in a staff house – a semi – in the school grounds. Such an arrangement was very convenient and meant that the staff had pastoral involvement with the patients as well as formal teaching positions. The staff enjoyed favourable rent levels in return.

"You see boys," said Mr. Wolfe to the group one day, "I could give Parsons here £1 with which he could go out and buy all the parts to build a bicycle and then sell it at a profit.

If I gave each of the rest of you £1 each, you would just end up with an odd assortment of components – I doubt that you could make one complete bicycle as a group. But Parsons, well, he has a gift to buy the right pieces at the right prices, and build a bike for a £1."

*

"It's stupid, going to church every Sunday."

"The vicar at St John's is Ok, just don't get into an argument with him."

"What a waste of a nice morning. I'd rather go walking across the fields instead of going to the Church. Still that mag was fun."

"Yeh, I've never seen Carrington go ballistic like that. Simon was shaking, just 'cos he'd picked up a QT mag from the pavement on the way to church. Wouldn't have taken it in would he?"

"Stupid it was. Couldn't see him hiding that behind a hymn book."

"Don't look at pictures, meet real girls" the Boss says. "It's all very well for him to say that – he's got a wife at home, he gets his end away – well, he is old mind, at least thirty – prob'ly past it.

'Sides which, those QT mags are stupid, no wonder someone threw it away. The girls in the pictures don't have nothing between their legs, no hair, no fanny, nothing. They don't show them because if they do then you get a raging horn and can't control yourself. Some of the boys don't believe that girls have got anything there at all. Even that girl at Nurse Hill's had one. It's not real – they must be covering it up with makeup or something."

"Don't be daft, you can't cover hair with makeup. You cover hair with a hat."

"You are mental! A girl with a hat between her legs! That's right silly that is! Huh! You're a flaming nutter! Anyway it's Monday tomorrow. Parsons will be back from his home visit. He's too clever by half. Surprised his father hasn't caught him nicking 'Spick and Spans' from the top shelf of the shop. If Carrington found out he was selling them here there'd be real trouble."

"Old Wolfey thinks the sun shines out of Parsons's arse."

"Yeh. Maybe his Father lets him sell the Spick and Spans?"

"P'raps. Wolfey said he was clever like that – got a knack for making money. Anyway, what can they do with him if they catch him here – they can't send him anywhere else, can they?"

"They could send him to Borstal or an Approved School."

"Nah, you get that for using a flick knife or a bicycle chain on somebody, like them Mods an' Rockers do down at Brighton. Or nicking stuff. Serious. Not for pinching apples or Spick an' Spans."

"They could search him when he comes back."

"Yeh, Carrington could start collecting the mags."

"Like oil! He's not like that."

"Maybe he's got a stash under his bed."

"Yeh, can you see Mrs. Carrington letting that happen? Like I said, he's prob'ly past it anyway."

"Flaming hell, I don't care about the Boss, what about me? How can anyone meet girls here? In church? Christmas party once a year. Ha! They don't even have dances in Boxmoor – everyone goes into Hemel or Hatfield on a Friday and Saturday. Or Top Ranking in Watford if they've got the dough. No flicks either."

"You can't meet girls in the flicks – it's dark, and you're in a seat. Top Ranking is much better. Smooching there. Great music too – The Beatles, Cliff Richard. You can even dance there on a Saturday morning."

"Well Simmsy said he met a girl at the flicks one Saturday, when he was home for the weekend. His stepdad gave him a pound to get rid of him, and he met some girls in the queue outside the Odeon."

"Never!"

"Yeh, sat with them right through the film he did."

"What – one on each hand, like?"

"Said he had a feel, but he would say that wouldn't he? Stands to reason he's not going to say that he sat with them all night and didn't get anything. We'd laugh at him. Well the others would anyway. I wouldn't."

"S'pose so. What film was it anyway?"

"Psycho something he said. By some bloke Hiscock."

"Psycho, Hiscock? Simmsy's 'aving you on! Nobody's called Hiscock!"

"Something like that it was. He said it was really scary and the girls wanted to hold his hand. An 'X' it was too."

"How'd he get in then? He don't look eighteen."

"Dunno, but he says he saw it. Girls were scared and screaming he said, wanted to hold his hand an' all, in fact everyone was screaming and jumping. Some woman gets stabbed and stabbed in the shower and there's a dead old woman in a chair an' all."

"Brilliant! Have to remember that – taking a girl to see a horror film."

"Yeh. Simmsy reckons that getting frightened softens 'em up, like. Putty in his hands he said. One even bought him an ice cream tub."

"Aw, brilliant!"

"Says the 'Pitting Pendulum' is on next week and he's going to see it. Same girls, too, he's goin' with. Real gory he said, loads of blood. He saw the trailer last week. Fancies one of them girls too. Gloria he said. Wouldn't say any more about her, though. Secret he says. Huh!"

"Pitting Pendulum? What's that about then?"

"Simmsy said it was a big axe swinging on a rope – cuts a woman in half – slowly."

"Wow, I bet that's something to see."

"Yeh, I bet. Anyway, I'm not going to the flicks, I'm not meeting any girls, and I can't remember when I last had a kiss, let alone a feel. Going to the Top Rank would be a dream."

"Don't worry, there's weekends at home, an' next year you'll be living at home."

"Like oil I will! I'm getting a place of my own. Susan's at home every night since she started in her secretarial course in Dacorum College. I'm not going near there to hear her go on about how she hates me. Maybe I'll call in and see Mum now an' again, when Susan's at college. She tells all her friends I'm mental, so there's no chance with Briony. No point being at home."

*

At Boxmoor, Susan's brother began to make progress with essential life skills. The teaching was supportive of the boys' individual interests.

The regime was relatively relaxed, and instrumental in equipping the patients (within their capabilities) for adult life. By the age of 11, in 1959, Susan's brother had a reading age of a 6 year old. By the time he was 13 in 1961, his reading and writing was good enough to support his technical interests – there is little that is more technical than amateur radio (at least in the 'everyday') – so he had made great advances.

Despite his emotional problems and slow academic development, Susan's brother began to catch up socially, as well as academically. Many others, though, never caught up. Many would end up in prisons, mental hospitals or early graves. The unnatural deaths resulted from high spirits – such as playing chicken with motorbikes – and all the other causes typical of this cohort, such as drugs overdoses, fights, stabbings and alcohol abuse.

*

There was some sexual experimentation by the boys – not at all unusual in a boarding environment with boys reaching puberty changing physically and becoming aware of sexual feelings for the first time. Susan's brother said 'no' to any involvement. His mind was firmly on girls.

"Steve said he fancied you."
"I'm not interested in any of that stuff."
"'Prob'ly best to keep away."
"You can say that again. I'd like a girlfriend some day. Some of the others say that they've done all sorts with girls. Maybe they have but I'm more interested in radio right now. Anyway, no girl is going to look at me. I'm ugly. I'll be lucky ever to have a girlfriend."
"Remember Dennis? He liked you."
"Grown-ups always tell lies. He was a bloke, in case you hadn't noticed. At least he made me laugh, even if he lied about South Africa. I'm not doing anything with men at all. Never have and

never will. Grown-ups always let me down. It's a girlfriend I'd like, or a better ham receiver – I really fancy an AR88."

*

Generally, he was enjoying his stay at Boxmoor and his emotional strength was building. However, as he had lacked affection from adults all his life, the gradual improvement in his self-esteem and confidence was painfully slow. But there was progress.

Until he arrived at the school, adults had seen him either as a problem to be solved, or a problem to be shunted elsewhere. Epping House had radical approaches, but couldn't stop the downward spiral to the suicide attempt.

At Boxmoor, R. A. Carrington, Mr. Wolfe and many of the other staff, recognised that, hidden within him, there was potential.

When he was at home during holidays, he used his transistor radio and would drop in to Gilbert & Co, the radio shop on Kings Road in Berkhamsted. Over several visits, Susan's brother got to know some of the staff in the shop, and asked them for a radio. They gave him a scrap valve 'wireless' which he took home with great delight.

Excitement was running high. First the crystal set, then a transistor radio, and now this scrap radio.

"How will you get it working?"

"I'll put up an aerial. Then, we'll see if we can get a signal. That Gerry Ayres is a tosser!"

"Well, Mum did say you had to get permission from the neighbours before you put up the aerial."

"What's Mr. Ayres so worked up about anyway. It's only a piece of four by four. I've saved the money for the wood, and now Gerry says 'No'. Huh. Make the road look like a council estate, he says. I'm doing it anyway. Bugger him."

Susan's brother brought home a 20 feet long length of wood – 4" x 4", solid and heavy – and erected it at the end of the garden, so that a proper aerial could be strung up for the new radio.

"He thinks it's 'unsightly'."

"Looks all right to me."

"Well, he's been moaning to Mum about it again."

"What're you going to do?"

"Nothing. Mum hasn't said anything to me since I put it up."

"It's funny."

"What?"

"Well, some of the neighbours moan about the aerial – Gerry Ayres 'specially – but Mum doesn't mind."

"Yeh, funny that. You'd think she'd stop me if the neighbours complained. Why do grown-ups always moan about stuff, and tell lies too."

"Search me."

The salvaged radio, with its long aerial worked, and one night, he heard some radio amateurs ('hams') talking on the 80m band (80 metres being the wavelength of the radio signal).

The language was mysterious.

What was CQ? What was signal strength? What did 5 by 5 mean? And 5 by 9? Where were these people talking from?

This was all new and exciting.

He phoned Uncle Frank, who had given him the ex-RAF headphones, and asked about what he'd heard. With Uncle Frank's help and encouragement he started to learn about the different wavelengths and the 'radio ham' world.

Finding out what the pupil's interests are, and stimulating the desire to learn from within the pupil, are fundamental aspects of effective education. Unfortunately, that process requires a lot of initial input and high staff/pupil ratios. Susan's brother was fortunate in that he was learning in an environment where close observation was both possible because of the high staff/student ratios, and essential because of the need to monitor the emotional health of the coterie.

His emotional development was progressing, the commitment of R. A. Carrington to teach him to think for himself was bearing fruit, and his introspection was becoming constructive. He was becoming less introverted as he started to form durable friendships.

Empathy was never lacking – certainly he'd felt sorry that his sister had to endure a brother who was a fat, ugly moron, but now he was beginning to turn empathy to positive use for social interaction.

The deep, nagging grudge he'd held against Mel Perkins at Epping House for saving his life had softened, and he began to understand another view of the event.

"They say I have to go home every weekend."

"Well, you are 13 now."

"I suppose so. Mother is not so bad to me now, Uncle Frank and Aunty Brenda have been visiting her a lot - maybe they have talked to her about you. She has had a tough time, losing Father, then your special schooling."

"Yes, but she treats Susan really well. You know how it is - she loves Susan but not me."

"Maybe she doesn't know how to love you, you are a boy. You don't play with dolls."

"No, and I was never allowed to have soft toys, except you."

"Girls and boys. Different - remember Nurse Hill?"

"Yeh, but I don't see what difference that makes. I feel sorry for Mother because she doesn't love me, she doesn't want me and thinks I'm useless. That's why I'm here, not because I miss Father like everyone says. Anyway, I played with you when you were around back at Dell Field Close."

"That was a long time ago. You can't carry a teddy bear around anymore."

"Father never let me carry you around, Ted."

"I know, but I did stay in your room."

"And Father beat you."

"You mustn't think badly of your father."

"I don't, but I *was* frightened of him."

"Yes. And your mother isn't perfect either. Maybe Father would have balanced things up if he was here. As I said, maybe Uncle

Frank and Aunty Brenda have helped her understand, and that's why she seems a bit nicer towards you."

"I suppose so, but Father's *not* here is he? At least Susan won't be there every weekend when I go home. I can't stand her going on about God and then hating me. Doesn't make sense at all. All that religious stuff she spouts - it makes me sick!"

Susan was now 15 years old. When she was about 13, she had 'got religion', and since then had been a regular churchgoer and had outwardly become increasingly righteous and God fearing. She often said that she saw her brother as a punishment which God had meted out to her, and she didn't know why she was being punished.

She gradually stopped telling her friends that her brother was mentally ill but Briony and Diana both knew him and had formed their own opinions. When they happened to be alone together, though – something her brother tried very hard to avoid – she let loose with her tongue and the cruel words were repeated.

*

In 1960, Susan's brother found his father's old bike in the garage and cleaned it up having outgrown his own bike.

"I'm going on a bike ride."

"Where?"

"To see Mel Perkins."

"But you hate him."

"Not any more. I was wrong to hate him for saving my life."

"Why do you want to see him?"

"I'm going to try to say I'm sorry."

"That's good."

"I think so."

"How far is it?"

"South Park Gardens to Epping House? It's about twenty eight miles, each way. Have you forgotten that I walked it twice when I ran away?"

"Oh yeh. That's a long way - I remember the walking."

"I'll be okay."

"Let's hope they let you in to see him, and that he will see you."

The trip up the A41 was a ride that no fourteen year old boy would be allowed to make today, unless with a cycling club. His mother certainly didn't know, but in those days of the late 1950's a young teenage boy disappearing for half a day was commonplace and no cause for concern.

When he arrived in Epping House, Mel Perkins was astounded to see him, and amazed that he'd made such a long journey on his bike.

"Two years is a long time. Your letter really upset him. He was only trying to save your life."

"I know, but I was really angry."

"I told you not to send it."

"Yeh, but it was good to talk to him about that night, and about what I felt."

"Did you understand his point of view, then?"

"Yes, I think he really did care about me."

"He was glad to hear you say Sorry?"

"I know, I'm glad I said it. It makes me feel much better."

*

As the months in Boxmoor House passed, Peter B started going to visit Susan's brother in South Park Gardens on the weekends – Susan's brother was only boarding at Boxmoor during the week. Peter would cycle over, and later came on his new motorbike. Mother liked Peter, and he enjoyed his time there, much more than he would have done with his own family. He was always greeted with a kiss on the cheek by Mother, who fussed over him – just as she had done with Nick Gynishe. These affectionate greetings were something that Susan's brother could not understand, and never received himself, though other school friends did on the very rare occasions that they visited – there were few of them.

Peter shared his interest in ham radio, and when there are two enthusiasts, learning is always easier and quicker as ideas are exchanged and problems puzzled out with two brains.

*

"It's funny, they don't do much religion at Boxmoor, except church on Sundays.

"Just as well – remember how you pissed off the vicar at Victoria School?"

"Yeh, that got me into trouble. Susan's gone all religious now, keeps saying I'm God's punishment to her."

"For what? What has she done wrong 'cept treat you badly?"

"'Dunno."

"Well, it's no surprise she's gone religious. She always was a bit funny. As far as she's concerned, everything is someone else's fault."

"You're right on that, but I'm fed up of hearing her asking why God has punished her by giving her a fat, ugly brother who can't read or write and will not get anywhere in life. She's so cruel to me, yet I'm sorry for her, having me as a brother."

"Well, you shouldn't be sorry, and you can read and write now. The tests they give you here prove it. You are making good progress."

"I can see that, but it doesn't stop Susan putting me down all the time. Sisters and brothers are supposed to love each other aren't they?"

"Yes in normal families."

"Well we can't be normal then."

*

In 1960, with his interest in radio developing strongly, and spending pocket money on Practical Wireless magazines, Susan's brother had saved up almost enough money from his Boxmoor House allowance, but was still short.

Susan's brother had his birthday in December, and as with many December- or January-born children, birthday and Christmas presents often get rolled together. That year, unusually, his family chipped in, with his mother, aunt and granny adding £10 as a joint birthday and Christmas present to buy another wireless on which he had set his sights. This very desirable radio was a serious piece of equipment – an ex-RAF R1155 receiver.

It was December, and he caught the train from Berkhamsted into London Euston. The shop was on Grays Inn Road, and Susan's brother carried the heavy, cumbersome, wartime radio set home.

*

By now he was a regular visitor to Gilbert & Co, and an assistant there told him about the Radio Society of Great Britain. The RSGB is the club for radio hams, and is responsible for ensuring the standards of technical proficiency of 'Radio Amateurs'. It was illegal for a radio amateur (or anyone else) to transmit unless they were licensed, and even then they had to transmit their call signs and were restricted to an output power of 150 watts. It doesn't sound much (1½ lightbulbs), but in the hands of an expert with the right equipment and at the right time of day, it is enough to talk to hams in Argentina or Australia, Canada or Australia. Although known as 'radio amateurs', some of these highly technical hams can bounce signals off the moon, download satellite weather maps direct from satellites, and carry out leading edge research. 'Amateur' really is a misnomer for many members of the Society.

*

Joining the RSGB led to Susan's brother developing social relationships outside Boxmoor House. The magazine 'Practical Wireless' had a personal ads column where radio hams sought penfriends. It was quite healthy. Nowadays, outside school, adolescents make friends on the web - on forums and bulletin boards, in chat rooms and on Facebook, with Twitter. These are all new channels for friendship (and bullying and abuse too), but many still make friends (as they did in 1960) through sports clubs – football teams, judo clubs, swimming clubs and 'youth clubs'. Susan's brother was no sportsman, clearly having difficulty catching a ball, given very poor hand/eye coordination.

In the early 1960s, when email was virtually undreamed of, youngsters had to write letters longhand and post them. There was no instant gratification or quick friendship. Letters took time – time to pen and time to post, and it might take four or five days to receive a reply, even from a nearby town.

Susan's brother developed a pen-friendship with Keith Lacock, who lived in Bradford. Susan's brother joined Chesham Amateur Radio Club and cycled there to the weekly meetings where he would meet other radio amateurs. His social circle widened.

By this time, he had learned about the 'ham exam' – the exam that he would have to pass if he was to become a qualified Radio Amateur, or 'Ham'. It is a technical exam, and requires knowledge of mathematics, electronics, physics (even of the earth's atmosphere and sunspots), and this was way beyond his formal level of education.

One of the members of the Chesham RSGB branch took an interest in Susan's brother and started to coach him to sit the Radio Amateur Examination.

"They were really mad, really cross about it."

"Yeh, wish I'd seen it."

"Who is this Hancock bloke?"

"Some sort of comedian, miserable bloke they said."

"How can anyone be miserable and a comedian?"

"Dunno, sounds daft to me."

"And he was making fun of Radio Amateurs?"

"Yeh. They didn't like his radio procedure, his call sign 'GLK' was wrong, his rig was just bits and pieces of old BBC studio junk. They hated it – a load of rubbish. Made them look like idiots, they said. And not only Hams, but he's made fun of Test Pilots too!"

"Never, not Test Pilots! Uncle Frank and Val would be cross about that."

"Maybe Bob Tolhurst watches this Hancock fellow?"

"Dunno, I'll ask him next week."

When Susan's brother was a boy, he was considered 'thick', stupid, slow and backward. Yes, he was technically backward in relation to the reading and writing capabilities of his peers, but had an enquiring mind, nevertheless. Uncle Frank had seen that, and fanned the spark. Others did their bit too, because they could see higher than average intelligence inside the sad, lonely and socially awkward lad. He may have been introverted, but he had a clear interest in the world around him.

They were a mixed crowd at the Radio Club and one member took a particular (and innocent) interest in him.

Alf is recalled as 'a hero', and provided Susan's brother with the technical explanation and support to sit the Radio Amateur Examination. Over the course of a year, cycling weekly to Alf's council house in Chesham, Susan's brother absorbed the jargon, the theory and the mathematics. This was a boy who was capable with his hands – he could build a rabbit hutch, take hide and stitch a wallet together, or assemble a transistor radio. This was a boy who had been considered disturbed, who had been measured as educationally subnormal, who had next to zero self-esteem, who had been bullied and ridiculed within his family, and without.

This boy was now being coached to use his brain, remember technical information and calculate using the speed of light as a constant. Beyond that, he would have to sit in a room, at a desk, recall that information, explain and apply the theory using the correct equations and calculate the results, writing in longhand. All done without books, without help, relying on his own brain, for two hours of what many would consider to be well above an 'O' level standard examination.

The building of sufficient confidence for him to go into the 'City and Guilds' exam at Luton Technical College, and of the belief that he actually might pass, was a major step forward for him.

The 'Tech' was 15 miles from home, and he cycled there and back for the exam, on a dark December evening. An exhausting bicycle ride before an examination is hardly something that would be thought sensible in modern times.

*

R. A. Carrington, the headmaster at Boxmoor, showed a real concern for Susan's brother, and was one of the few people ever to ask him whether he was 'OK'. At lunchtimes during the week, Susan's brother sat on the same dining table as Mr. Carrington.

This apparent favouritism did not result in any adverse reaction from the other boys – as at Beech House, the boys had five minutes to eat their meals before the plate was removed – that was the rule, although it was not rigidly enforced. So, there was little time for chatter, the focus was on finishing the food within the allotted time.

One day there was conversation, and it is remembered still. Unusually, it originated from Susan's brother.

"That was brave."

"What?"

"Asking Mr. Carrington if you are maladjusted."

"Not brave. I need to know, see, and I can talk to him. He treats me like I'm normal."

"Yeh, well now you know you're normal."

"Yep, I'm glad I asked. 'No', he said, 'not maladjusted. You are just behind with your education'."

"What's maladjusted mean?"

"Dunno."

"Everyone here uses the word though."

"At least you're not."

"Not what?"

"Maladjusted."

"Yeh, whatever that is. Sounds like a clock that's gone wrong."

"Brilliant though!"

"Yeh brilliant. I wonder what Susan would say."

"Prob'ly something cruel."

"Yeh, prob'ly."

"And Mum?"

"Prob'ly nothing, she wouldn't say anything."

"What do you think about Mr. Carrington's shotgun then?"

"Brilliant! He really knows how to use it."

"Yeh, what with the foxes trying to get at his chickens and eggs. But seeing in the dark like that!"

"I couldn't see bugger all – it was pitch black."

"He's got eyes like an owl, seeing in the dark like that. I heard he was in the war in the desert, fighting the Germans. Desert Rats or something."

"Wow! Wonder how many he killed?"

"Prob'ly loads, eyes like that, and a good shot too. It was great for him to take me and Parsons out last night. I didn't know what was going to happen. Then those flashes, and the noise - wow!"

"Yeh, I don't know how he could see those rats and hit them like that."

"Weren't much left of them this morning."

"No. Must have scared the Germans in the war, being able to shoot in the dark like that."

"I'll bet he did!"

*

There were escapades and diversions, some serious and some amusing – just part of life in a school full of energetic (though disturbed) boys.

In 1961, there was an emergency resulting from an attempted prank. In the grounds, one of the oak trees was set up with a rope, as a swing. John C had the idea to untie the rope from the oak and reattach with a piece of string. He kept this to himself, and one evening set the prank and went back to the dining room for supper.

The next day, John went out into the grounds and forgetting the prank, he went to the swing. He spent the next month unconscious in hospital, but eventually recovered from the coma.

*

Back at South Park Gardens, Mrs. Robinson was still working at TAM. At home, she passed her time reading and sewing. Books came from the public library and at least one thriller was always present on the coffee table alongside a copy of the Daily Mail. Mother did not read Mills and Boon. There were occasional cinema trips with Mrs. Malet, with whom she had worked at Ashlyns School. Mrs. Malet was relatively high-brow and considered herself to be a film buff. There were regular discussions in South Park Gardens about films, though TV was starting to make inroads into the general public consciousness. Coronation Street was barely a year old, and the whole concept of 'soaps' was unknown to the British public. In 1960, TV as a form of entertainment was still somewhat tacky in the eyes of the English middle class.

She was very particular about her appearance, having her hair done regularly, and always being smartly turned out, though there had been, apparently, no male interest in her life. It seemed that Robbo had meant everything to her, and there would be no replacement.

That year, on her birthday, Susan's brother clubbed together with Peter B and they bought her a top-of-the-range Russell Hobbs electric kettle. It was vastly superior to the old gas kettle, and she was delighted with the gift.

*

"I'm still a problem for her."

"Why, how?

"Well now I'm at home on weekends, the neighbours see me."

"So? They know you anyway."

"Yes, but did you hear what Susan said?"

"What?"

"She said:"

"Oh, you're home now. I suppose I'll have to tell the neighbours that you are mentally ill."

"That's not very nice."

"Well, I suppose it's true."

"Not."

"Is."

"Grow up!"

"Mum hardly ever asks me how I am."

"Does it matter?"

"Yes it matters. It would be nice to think she was interested if I was well or not, how things were here, you know, like she cared a bit. She liked the electric kettle, though it was Peter who got the hug, as if I had no part in it."

*

"Phew! She's a bit of all right!"

"Yeh, those stringy black dresses really make her look good. For a social worker or whatever she is. Coming to school dressed like that. Someone nice to think about before I go to sleep."

"Yeh, and she really drives that Hillman Minx with a bit of go."

"You said it, she's got something, all right. Miss Asher is the sort of woman I'd like to have as a girlfriend."

"Don't be daft – she's ten years older than you!"

"No, you're being daft, when I'm older I mean. Still, I'd take it now if it was on offer."

"Well, it's not. She's probably got loads of blokes buzzing around her like bees round a honeypot."

"Yeh, well I can dream can't I? And we're all malads here anyway."

"Prob'ly right there. Bet she can have anyone."

"I'm going to sleep now."

"Sweet dreams."

"Shut up!"

*

All through his years at Boxmoor, there were regular meetings with Miss Asher, the psychiatric social worker who had been assigned Susan's brother as part of her caseload. The discussions were relatively informal as she sought to 'open up' the boy and get him to talk. There was a series of core questions at the heart of the meetings and, no doubt, a structure into which the responses were slotted so that progress (or otherwise) could be measured.

There is no recollection of the final meeting, but certainly there would have been a point at which a final assessment had been recorded, and the decision made that Susan's brother could be released to play his part in the normal world. He would not be going on to a more senior institution for the mentally disturbed.

After his 14th birthday in 1961, the staff thought that Susan's brother was ready to live at home, and be a day pupil at Boxmoor House. He was maturing, his confidence was improving, and the last two years' weekends at home had been moderately successful in re-integrating him into home life.

"Blimey, Mum didn't know what to say."

"Well she doesn't talk to me much anyway."

"Reckon she was worried when she saw that blue 'City and Guilds' crest on the envelope."

"Prob'ly thought it was something official about me."

"Well it was."

"No, doctors or school or something, you know what I mean."

"Yeh. She seemed a bit surprised you'd passed."

"Bet she never thought she'd see the day I passed an exam."

"Are you going to tell Susan?"

"No."

"Oh. Who then?"

"Well, Alf – I owe a lot to him, and the boys over at Chesham radio club. Oh – and I might phone Mr. Carrington tonight."

*

The next morning, at assembly in Boxmoor, Mr. Carrington announced briefly, with no flourish, that Susan's brother had passed the City and Guilds Radio Amateur Examination. Peter B had left for the day school at Apsley Grammar, and he was the only Boxmoor boy who had any idea what the exam was.

*

Six months after he had bought the R1155 ex-RAF receiver, Susan's brother bought the companion transmitter, the T1154. He was still a virgin, in the heterosexual sense.

"It's busy."

"Yeh, well it's Saturday."

"I bet Tottenham Court Road is busy every day."

"'Prob'ly. Look at all that gear. Radio shops everywhere."

"I've never seen so many radiograms and tape recorders. And some of that Ferrograph gear. I wish I could one of those to tape the radio traffic."

"Maybe one day."

"Yeh, one day, maybe."

"Yeh. This T1154 is killing me though. So heavy."

"It's not far to Euston now."

"Yeh, but if I drop it or bump it then the valves might get damaged. I've got to take a breather – look there's a bench."

"That man in Henry's Radio was really helpful."

"No wonder - I'll bet he was glad to get rid of it – these transmitters are a bit past it now. People don't want to wait for the 807s to warm up. Transistors are the thing."

"807s?"

"Valves you berk. They take 5 minutes to warm up, and you've got to watch the colour so they don't overheat. If they get blue you'll strip the cathode."

"Blue? Strip Cathy's wot's it?"

"Berk! Damage the valve. Strip the cathode."

"Oh, technical. I thought that was going to be interesting then, 'bout some girl called Cathy. That reminds me. What was all that about with that girl before we went into Henry's? Any idea what she was prattling on about?"

"No idea. 'Did I want a good time'? Don't know what she was on about. Silly cow. What business could I do with her?"

"Nice looking though."

"Yeh, bit tarty, mind, went on a bit. Not as nice as Diana."

"Are you still keen on her then?"

"Not half. It's a pity she's so friendly with Susan."

"Oh, staying away from her then, are you? One day you'll have a fully transistorized rig, but still be a virgin."

"Huh it's looking that way! An AR88 would be nice, but my first proper girlfriend would be even better."

*

Sid Coombes was an occasional weekend visitor to South Park Gardens.

"I'm going to have to make the desk bigger."

"Maybe Sid will come back another weekend and help you extend it."

"Pr'aps, I'll have to ask Mum. If he does, I'll need money to buy more blockboard. Till then it's going on the floor."

"Won't it stack on the R1155?"

"I'll try it."

"What do you think Susan will say?"

"Dunno, but probably something cruel. It's going to be worse now she goes to the Tech to do that secretary's course, living at home. Says she's to trying do it in one year. Everyone else takes two. A right clever so-and-so, she is.

I'll go nuts with her being at home in the evenings and at weekends, and she won't be too happy either, having her mental brother there when she brings her friends home. Still, I'll shut myself in my room, and have the T1154 and R1155 side by side, and the door locked."

"You'll 'go nuts' – that's a funny one coming from you. At least she'll be bringing her friends there – Diana and the others. You'll get to see them. Diana doesn't think you're mental."

"Maybe."

"Ok. Anyway, what are you going to use the T1154 for – you haven't got a licence to transmit?"

"Yeh, and no chance of getting one either - I still can't make head or tail of the Morse Code. The T1154 only cost a quid though, so I'll use it for parts. Then maybe one day I'll have a full transistorized rig, and pass my Morse exam. Not much hope of that, though. I just can't do the Morse code by ear. Five words a minute! I can't even do one. Not even with a crib sheet."

Although he had passed the Radio Amateur Foundation Exam, he did not have a licence to transmit and could not obtain one. Such a licence would require passing a practical test in Morse Code transmission and 'reading' – decoding the stream of Morse dots and dashes as it was received through the radio. His brain couldn't process it.

*

Sid Coombes was working as an architect's assistant, living in digs, and Valerie would invite him over, recognising that he was a positive influence on Susan's brother. When he was visiting, he would take Susan's brother into town on a Saturday, and treat him.

"I got confused about that."

"Not half as confused as Sid was."

"Yeh, well, it was great of him to buy me that air pistol."

"Eventually."

"Yeh, I seem to get some words confused."

"You can say that again! He says to you 'Would you like an air pistol?' and you say ..."

"...yes, I know – 'I've got to insult my mother first'. I seem to get 'insult' and 'consult' mixed up. Other words too."

*

At the ham radio club in Chesham, one of the members was selling a motorbike. It was a BSA B31 single cylinder unit, and the price was £2. Susan's brother bought the bike with money he had saved, and spent weekend hours riding it around the building site. Another piece of technology had come into his life, albeit basic technology. However it was another interest pursued by an enquiring mind.

Unfortunately, the neighbours were not so understanding and apart from pointing out that he was only thirteen years old, they didn't like the noise nor did they like him racing up and down the building site that was the emerging North park Gardens.

He decided to dispose of the bike, and with a friend they pushed it into the Grand Union Canal. The choice of location was poor, and the canal was in those days heavily silted. The motorbike stood there, gaunt and erect, its handlebars above water.

"That was stupid."

"Yeh, didn't think to check the depth. It looked funny though, sitting there with the handlebars above water."

"The copper didn't think it was funny when he gave you the ticket. He was raving."

"The Beak didn't think it was funny either. Now you've got a fine and you'll have a record, too, I bet. You berk!"

"I don't have my motorbike, I've been fined for dumping - that's more of my pocket money gone – and now you're calling me a berk. I don't need it. You know – I'm glad you're not around so much these days."

"You need to think harder about what you do, not about radios, girls and motorbikes. You haven't got time to talk to me anymore."

"Ok, ok, I'm trying, right? Not jealous are you?"

"No, not jealous, it just means you don't need me so much 'cos you're getting better. Remember what Mr. Carrington said?"

"Yes, yes, he would teach me to think for myself."

"Well, bloody well start thinking then, and I'll keep out of the way."

"Ok, ok, no need to swear!"

*

"I'm learning a lot from Bob. I love having tea there, and he always makes the TV news seem interesting."

"You just go there to see Briony and dream about her."

"Get off! Bob explains the news. I always believed everything they said on TV. Now he makes me think about how they don't always tell the real truth. Grown-ups lying again."

"Yeh, helping you to think for yourself. Mr. Carrington said that too."

"Don't keep on about Mr. bloody Carrington!"

"Ok, cool down."

"Bob reads the Daily Telegraph too. That's a big paper – mostly words, not like the Daily Sketch, all pictures. He seems to know about everything, and what he doesn't know he can find out. That's smart. He loves his garden, too. I wonder why."

"Think about it. He likes to grow his own food."

"Why doesn't he keep pigs then, and make sausages?"

"You're being silly now."

"Don't know what a traffic engineer does, whatever that is, but when he gets home, he changes out of his suit and straight into his gardening clothes. Why go gardening and get dirty if you're a traffic engineer and wear a suit to work? Seems daft to me. He's always digging for supper. It's easier to buy it – he must have plenty of money for food."

"Well, maybe it's his hobby, like you have radio. He has his garden."

"Hadn't thought of it like that."

"Well, start using your brain a bit more. Some things you have to work at. Like you work at the radio, soldering and saving for your next rig, Bob digs. He and the others worked hard to persuade the Council about turning that land into allotments."

"S'pose so."

"You remember it - derelict, no use to anyone between the railway line and the back of the garden. You built your radio, and fiddle with it. He got his allotment and digs in it."

"Yeh, at least it's being put to some use now. But gardening though!"

"Some people may say that about train spotters, or even radio hams. And he's got three daughters to feed. That can't be cheap."

"Yeh, three daughters. Briony too. Ok, Ted that's enough for tonight. Just go to sleep, will you? I want to do some thinking of my own."

"Not Briony again?"

"Shut up and go to sleep!"

"'Night."

"'Night."

*

"That was a laugh."

"Peter though it was very funny!"

"It was!"

"Everyone in Apsley Gram knows, prob'ly in Boxmoor too. Prob'ly even all of Berkhamsted?

"Blimey, what a thought! It was James's own fault anyway – fancy trying to pull down a girl's knickers in school!"

"James is lucky to have girls in his school. Boys and men, that's all we've got here."

"Yeh, well, bad luck to be caught too."

"Yeh – he's not stupid, should have been more careful. Said Wrigley went nuts, said that Wrigley gave James a thrashing, then said it was 'unacceptable to do that in school but was all right at home.'"

"You've got to laugh. He doesn't know the half of it. Huh!"

"Yeh, she's a cracker all right."

"Better than Nurse Hill!"

"Loads better."

"You've got no chance there mate."

"I'm going to take my time, maybe things will be different one day."

*

"We've got new neighbours, moved in last week, at the end of the road. They've got a daughter, Susan. She's nice. Met her on the weekend."

"Talk to her did you?"

"Yeh, a bit. She was going to the shop for her Mum. I do like her. Trouble is, I'm only there on weekends."

"And holidays."

"Yeh, but the holidays are months away and I hate being there with Susan, she's always nasty. So I'm stuck here in the week, while she'll be getting to know Yatesey and the others in the street. I won't have a chance."

*

As spring turned to summer and the evenings lightened, Peter B, who was now once again living at his family home, became a regular visitor on Tuesday and Thursday evenings. He and Susan's brother spent increasing amounts of time together, sharing an interest in amateur radio. Peter, though, never sat the Radio Amateur examination.

On Sunday mornings, at home in South Park Gardens, Susan's brother would be tuning in his R1155 receiver - it was better than Family Favourites on the radio, which his mother and another five million people loved to listen to. One day, he picked up a broadcast by a ham, call sign G3EFP.

The signal-strength meter showed that the signal was very strong – suspiciously strong – and it looked as if the ham was putting out much more than the 150 watts legal maximum transmission power. Using the RSGB directory, Susan's brother was able to cross check the ham's call sign to find out the phone number; he called up the ham broadcaster whilst he was on air.

His name was Jack P, and he lived in a bungalow at the end of a lane in a nearby village.

He invited Susan's brother to visit and see his equipment. It was an AR88 receiver – the best in the world at the time, with a full length – 80 metre – dipole aerial strung out down his substantial garden.

Susan's brother became a regular visitor.

"Where's his wife? A forty year old man should have a wife."

"He hasn't got one. He's as bent as a nine bob note."

"Yes, but he's got a great transmitter. And a full length aerial too."

"I know, but he takes his clothes off."

"Well, I ignore that. He doesn't try anything on."

"So far. Don't you think it's wrong, him doing that when you are there?"

"He just likes to do everything with no clothes on. I don't mind it - I don't know if it's right or wrong. I'd run a mile if he tried anything. He's nice, and he always buys Lyons Fruit Pies. He actually asks what flavour I'd like! Not many people care about me like that. I've always had to eat what I've been given, no choice."

"He's involved with the Boy Scout movement."

"Yes, he's even got a copy of Baden Powell's "Scouting for Boys" on his bookshelf."

"I bet he does a lot of that."

"What – put books on his shelf?"

"No. Scouting for boys."

"You reckon?"

"Yeh, I do – he sounds weird."

"I've only just had my first real kiss, and girls really do get me going, make me feel different inside. I just don't understand queers."

"What about Nurse Hill, eh? Remember that?"

"Yeh, Nurse Hill. Can we talk about something else?"

"You're in charge, it's your brain, you berk."

"What do you reckon on Jack's car then?"

"Brilliant, though it's not modern like a Cortina or a Mini."

"Daimler Dart, V8, drop head. I'd love one."

"I'm not sure about the colour though. It's poncy. I'd want a red one. I wonder if it's got more poke than a Zodiac."

"Dunno, definitely more than a Mini though, or an Anglia. Maybe I'll have one, one day."

"Yeh, and pigs may fly. It would be really groovy though, my own sports car – a red one. Might have a chance with some girls then."

*

"Good party – the music was great, don't know what they'd have done without you."

"Yeh. Trouble is that there weren't many records and most of them were old anyway."

"Twenty five watts isn't much for an amplifier at a dance."

"A dance? That wasn't a dance. Dances are regular things, not once a year. That was a Christmas party – sort of. Who wants a party with the teachers there? Can't do anything."

"I know, but – well, you know – they're not too bad, and at least they invited some of the local girls in."

"Yeh, but what's the point of meeting girls once a year? Meet girls they say. How can we do that? I'm not dancing with boys the rest of the time."

"Fair enough, but that Babs really fancied you – see the way she was looking at you?"

"Huh! I was getting on great, thought things were going to go somewhere, y'know?"

"Yeh, so what happened then?"

"She let it slip – "

"Let what slip?"

"Shut up and let me finish! She said that she was oldest in the second year - she's only thirteen. Can't do nothing there can I? So what anyway, even if she was my age, when could I meet her? It's stupid. Next year, I'm going to ask Susan Tarry to come to the dance with me."

"Susan? Keen on her then, are you?"

"Not half! And she's not a friend of my sister. Just wait, next year I'll have Susan Tarry, more power in the amp, and a tape recorder too, with better music. If there wasn't so much fade, I'd put Radio Luxembourg on. It's much better late at night."

"Yeh, but they wouldn't let a party go on late."

"No, you're right, that's another daft thing. Maybe I could tape a couple of late shows from Radio Luxembourg."

"Maybe, but there's all those ads. You don't want Horace Batchelor and his football pools ads. 50 watts of 'K – E – Y – N – S – H – A – M, Bristol'. Everyone will be shouting it and stamping the floor."

"I could edit that out."

"How?"

"Splice the tape."

"What's that??

"Cut it and glue it"

"You can ac'shully do that for every advert?"

"Yeh, easy. It's what all the radio stations do. Same with film in the cinema too."

"Brilliant! Anyway, we won't be here next year."

"Oh yeh. Right strange that'll be. I wonder where I'll be living – not at home with Mother and Susan. I hope I can get a job and a place of my own. Have some girls round. A real Christmas party of my own. Lights out, some games and stuff, you know."

"Yeh, but you'll need to meet the girls first."

"It's got to be easier than it is here!"

"Yeh, got to be."

*

"He's going back to Libya."

"Where's that?"

"Africa I think. He does something in an oil company. In the desert."

"Must be more than delivering petrol if he has a car like that and an AR88 too."

"Yeh, he's dead clever, and he's really helped me with the radio stuff."

"And the fruit pies."

"Yeh, don't remind me. He's the only person who's ever asked me what pudding I'd like. It's been a brilliant summer, he's taught me a lot."

"Yeh, radio and fiddling about."

"No, I told you before, no fiddling – just radio."

"Okay, okay, cool down. Wonder what he'll do with his car?"

"Dunno, leave it here I suppose. They only have camels 'n stuff in the desert."

"Blimey. No roads?"

"Dunno. Sand mostly I 'spect."

"Yeh, can't be much fun."

"Dennis wanted you to go to Africa too."

"Don't remind me. What is it about Africa?"

"Dunno."

"Still, Jack gave me sixty feet of wire for an aerial. And there were always ciggies too. He was a great bloke with a great car and a great radio."

"Who liked doing transmitting in the nude."

"Yeh, weird."

*

"I think I'm in love."

"Love, you? I thought you didn't know what the word meant."

"Well, I've got this funny feeling."

"About who?"

"Susan."

"Susan, are you mad, she's your sister!"

"No, you berk. Susan Tarry."

"Ah, yes. Susan Tarry. Soft on her then are you?"

"Reckon so. She's gorgeous. And the way her petticoat holds her dress out like, like, well you know? I can see her now. Trouble is her Mum and Father are not keen on her going out with me."

"How do you know? You've been to her house haven't you?"

"Just a feeling I get. Being at a special school an' all. No wonder they're not keen."

"Have, they stopped her from seeing you?"

"No, not as far as I know."

"Well, ask Susan herself about it then."

"I'm afraid to do that, don't want to spoil anything. Anyway, doesn't matter really, as long as she can go on seeing me. She's my first proper girlfriend."

"What do you mean by 'proper'"

"Holding hands, walking together, kissing."

"Is that all? That's slow going if that's all you got. You had more luck with Katie."

"Katie was different, and Susan Tarry is different – I care about her.

"Care? I thought you didn't understand what it was."

"Well, I'm learning, got this funny feeling. Anyway, stop being nosy."

"You started talking about her first."

"It's because I can't stop thinking about her."

"You've really got it bad then you poor sod."

"Leave me alone, will you? I'm stopping now so mind your own business and shut up. I want to go to sleep."

"Fat chance of that, isn't there?"

*

"Mr. Carrington thinks I should try and work in radio. Maybe a TV engineer or something like that. He says I have an aptitude."

"Attitude about what?"

"I SAID APTITUDE YOU BERK!"

"Ok don't shout. People are looking at you. They'll think you're a nutter shouting in the street like that with no-one else there. They'll put you back inside again."

"I still mix my words up. They can't do that. Mr. Carrington reckons I'm ready. Mum still doesn't care though. And I'm fed up with the Morse lessons too. Mr. Carrington's mate is good at it, but even he can't teach me. I reckon my brain's not right for it. I'll never get the Amateur licence, and I'm going to give up trying. I don't know whether I can get a job as a radio engineer without Morse."

"Sure you can – there's always the TV anyway – no Morse code with that is there? And it's all the rage now. Selling like hot cakes they are. Radiograms too. Bush, Grundig – there's bound to be loads of jobs."

"Yeh, maybe."

"Yeh, for sure, it's the best thing for you. Look at all those other poor sods at Boxmoor – where are they going to end up?"

"Parsons will do ok, he's got a knack for making money."

"Yeh, but he's just one out of how many – a couple of dozen?"

"Where are they going to end up? Count your blessings and follow The Boss's advice. He knows what he's talking about."

"We'll see. I need to think about it."

*

Susan's brother had leapt forward in his education and confidence at Boxmoor.

What had made it effective for him and helped him succeed?

Was it the regime and the positive influence of the staff, or was it just maturity and healing?

His sister no longer belittled him in front of her friends, though she continued with her question about 'why God was punishing her with such a brother' in the rare accidental moments of being alone together.

Since Beech House and his altercation with Keith, he had not felt physically threatened, and had not been bullied so much. His growth had caught up with other of his age, and that had helped.

The strange respect which had started in Victoria School when he was called 'The Professor', was still there, and had grown as he mastered the complex hobby of amateur radio. His nickname now was 'Robbo', just as his Father's had been.

His interests in radio, motorbikes and the school go-kart were diverting his attention outward, and there was less time and energy left for introspection.

Years of being told that he was a fat, ugly moron with no future had hard-wired these ideas into his brain, and replaying the tapes when he was alone, and before going to sleep, reinforced those destructive mantras. Today, it would be called NLP – neuro-linguistic programming.

The environment at Boxmoor, the dedicated staff, his developing friendships and his hobbies, together with his improving emotional state, were now starting to erase those deeply laid tracks.

He was interested in girls, and started realise that they did not think he was fat and ugly, otherwise they would not go out with him.

"I'll never forget that. What a day."

"Yeh, she was magic."

"Perfect it was, like the films. Sunny, hot, lying there in the grass, Susan Tarry next to me. My first kiss. She tasted great, and her lips were so soft."

"What did she taste of – Sunday lunch?"

"Stop that you berk!"

"Hah! Next year the builders will have put a house on that spot."

"Yeh, thanks for reminding me, that field will never be the same again. I can still taste her mouth now."

"Go to sleep you dirty bugger."

"It's not dirty, it's lovely."

"Not what you are thinking!"

"Hey, I've got to start somewhere."

"Just go to sleep will you?"

*

First Steps from Boxmoor

"You are nearly fifteen now, Boxmoor will soon be in the past. Are you ready?"

"Ready for what?"

"Whatever comes next. You've made it through tough schools, ten years since your father dies. In and out of special homes, mixing with nutters. You've taken all that's been thrown at you and you're still in one piece. You've got two front teeth now, hobbies, skills, you've even had your first kiss, got your first girlfriend. The world is changing, fast.

You've got to make it on your own now. I can't help you much more. Besides, you don't need my help. I'll still be there though, sleeping. You can think for yourself. Mr. Carrington said he'd teach you that, if nothing else."

"He did."

"Well, what are you going to do with yourself?"

"The Boss said I should focus on radio. How am I going to do that?"

"Ask a friend."

"Who?"

"Bob Tolhurst. He understands how the world works. It's Monday, I'll talk to him tonight."

*

In December 1962, when he reached the age of fifteen, Susan's brother left Boxmoor. He had had (by his own choice) only minimal time at home, and socialisation with normal children had been minimal. After almost five years of close supervision and what passed for 'care', of interminable discussions with educational psychologists and child psychiatrists, the boy who had been described as severely disturbed and had lived for years in special schools, the boy who had spent two weeks in an adult male mental ward, was finally cast adrift into society.

The slow tapering-off of full time boarding to being a weekdays student, the interest of one or two perceptive teachers and his interaction with caring neighbours had all helped to prepare him for this major step change in his life.

However, Susan was still living at home and a difficult transition period was in prospect as he left Boxmoor on his last day.

*

Chatting to Bob Tolhurst was not especially helpful about the immediate future, beyond the practical encouragement and positive attitude that he fostered in the teenager.

At Chesham Amateur Radio Club however, things took a turn for the better. A club friend who had been trying patiently to teach him Morse Code, Tim Woodman, worked for a company called 'Rediffusion', which ran a chain of TV rental shops. They rented basic sets which were badged for them by TV manufacturers. Demand for television sets was snowballing. BBC colour television was still five years away, and in 1962 the cost of black and white sets was, in 2011 terms, close to £1,000. 'TV rental' was a rapidly growing market sector – many people couldn't afford to buy TVs outright or had difficulty buying them on hire purchase.

Rediffusion also specialised in cable relays for delivering radio and TV signals – schools television was another market they addressed – they were UK pioneers in what was ultimately to become cable TV. An associated company would later win the first commercial (ITV) license in the UK, for the London area.

As far as radio and television was concerned, the company was at the forefront of developments in 1962, in what was still, then, Great Britain.

Tim suggested that Susan's brother apply for an apprenticeship. After completing the application form, he attended two interviews and impressed Rediffusion with his electronics aptitude and the fact that he had passed the City & Guilds Radio Amateur Examination.

*

"I've got it!"
"Got what?"
"Rediffusion."
"Is that a disease?"
"No, an apprenticeship you fool!"

"What, Rediffusion - like those people who make TV programmes. Are you going to be on TV?"

"No, no, no. Stop messing about. It's an apprenticeship. They have a radio and TV division and they offered me one. I'm going to be an apprentice, learning how to repair TV sets."

"What's an apprentice?"

"Someone who signs a contract, and learns a trade 'on the job'"

"Sex you mean?"

"No! You are starting to wear me out now with stupid questions."

"Sorry. Got to have a laugh sometime. I'm you, remember?"

"Well, they learn the practical side of things working with skilled tradesmen, and one day a week they go to college and learn to pass exams. Then they get their trade."

"After how long?"

"I think it's at the age of 21."

"Blimey, that's six years!"

"Yeh, it's a long time."

"Why don't they go to college every day?"

"Because the trade is practical. It's not like a bank manager, sitting behind a desk all day with a pencil, getting fat on other people's money. It's fixing things."

"What, like unblocking his drains."

"That's plumbers, but you're getting the idea."

"What's 'Getting a Trade' mean then?"

"Well after passing the exams, so you know the theory stuff, and serving your time – no jokes – as an apprentice with qualified tradesmen, then you become qualified yourself."

"But you can fix radios. Why spend six years learning?"

"I need to learn about TVs too – they're big now, and colour TV will be here soon – it's in America now. Getting a trade is a qualification, right?"

"Oh. That's sounds good then."

"It is, but there's some bad news too."

"What?"

"That Caroline – Mrs. Tolhurst says I can't go out with her."

"Why not? She must be ok if she's a friend of Vivienne. And she's clever enough to go to Apsley Grammar."

"That's what I thought. How can she stop me?"

"No way, I suppose, but you listen to the Tolhursts, they talk sense."

"Yeh. I'll have to think on that."

"On Caroline?"

"Yeh, her too. I'm nuts on her. I want to take her to see 'Summer Holiday' next week, at the Empire in Hemel. She's nuts on Cliff Richard."

"She should be nuts on you!"

"Yeh, it's a funny world isn't it? And it's funny that Mrs. Tolhurst wants me to stay away from her, I don't know why. Probably they think I'm not good enough for her."

"Don't be daft, they really like you, treat as a normal human being."

"Maybe, but what other reason could there be?"

*

"I'm worried."

"What now, what's got you worked up today? If someone has threatened you then just thump him."

"It's not that. It's the Gower boys."

"What about them?"

"They've got some Danish girlie magazines."

"Wow, that's brilliant."

"They show the hair on the girls' fannies."

"Brilliant, but so what?"

"So what? So what is that I didn't get a raging horn and become uncontrollable, that's what."

"So?"

"Well I can't be normal then can I?"

"Why?"

"Well I though they didn't show the hair otherwise blokes would go wild. I saw the hair and I didn't go mad."

"That's daft."

"It's not."

"It is!"

"No, it can't be right, otherwise half the country would be mad, stands to reason. Practically every man with a wife would be going crazy every night."

"Maybe they do. I don't have a father so how would I know what goes on in a normal house at night."

"What about the Richard and Peter – they've got the mags – did they go mad?"

"No. Maybe they're not normal either."

"No, it's you it is, probably worrying about nothing. Ask them if their Dad goes mad at night."

"Maybe women cover themselves, to stop men going mad like that."

"Maybe some do, but I think you are making a mountain out of a molehill. Ask Peter and Richard."

"OK. They were good mags though. And now I think about the pictures, I do feel a bit funny."

"Go to sleep."

"I'll try. But those pictures are on my mind."

*

"Brilliant, I got the letter! I start on 1 October at the Training Centre. They say I'll be going to the Tech' one day a week too."

"Where will you live?"

"Probably Greenford. I'll have to find digs – get a local paper and start looking. Bob Tolhurst was really pleased for me!"

"Did you find out why they didn't want you to go out with Caroline?"

"No. I'm going to look for someone else and forget about her. They must be right, though I don't know why."

*

The apprenticeship at Rediffusion started straight after he left Boxmoor in December 1962. He found digs in Lady Margaret Road in Southall. The landlady was a homely Irishwoman who treated him just as she treated the other lodgers of his age – not special, not different, just normal. It was a completely new experience for him. He lived there during his first year whilst studying at Perivale Government Training Centre. At the same time he attended Southall Technical College where he studied City & Guilds 2nd Radio and TV Servicing. He bought another motorbike and suffered his fair share of the usual practical jokes typical dished out to teenagers in their first job.

Susan's brother was still relatively naïve, although his trust in adults was low which countered that to an extent. So, he couldn't be persuaded to 'go to the stores and ask for a tin of elbow grease'. Practical jokes were something that he couldn't play a part in, although he had deceived people himself – for example, his mother over the weekly Cubs visits that rarely took place.

He was now riding a BSA C11G motorbike, but after six months of use, the gearbox had failed.

"How will you get to work now?"

"Steve Balchin said he'd lend me his Bantam."

"That's decent of him."

"Yeh."

Steve Balchin was a neighbour in South Park Gardens, and used a car for commuting. He'd heard about the predicament and helped out with the loan of his BSA Bantam motorbike. It was a valuable favour, which went unappreciated. The episode was not forgotten, though.

"He wasn't happy about that."

"Don't remind me. He said that there was a bolt missing from the engine and that the bike was dirty. Said I hadn't looked after it properly."

"Well, he's right."

"Yeh. I did nothing to it in three months – just put petrol in. He did me a good favour, and I let him down."

"Learn from it then!"

"Don't worry, I will."

*

The Driving Test

Erections arrive earlier these days, as puberty occurs earlier – a consequence of better nourishment and social pressure, but an adolescent boy knows that ejaculation does not make him a man. There are other measures such as chest hair and pubic hair that are used for comparison in the showers. Beyond the body, there are external measures too.

The first car in a young man's life is never forgotten. For many, it is the one thing that finally convinces them that they are men. For others, it is the first legal pint of ale in a pub. Nowadays, both events are legalised at the same age of 18. Both 'comings of age' are not healthy when taken together. 18 is also the legal 'age of majority' when a young man (or woman) may vote. Neither was necessary to die for Queen and Country in the 1960's (and continues today, though not directly for armed operations).

16 was the age then, and still is – and for sexual intercourse too. It's strange that for events which involve putting one's life at risk for the State, or creating life itself, one does not have to be an adult in the legal sense, at least in the United Kingdom. The opportunity to vote at 18 is of no consequence to many young men of 18, there are other things which are much more important. It may be that first full sexual encounter or it may be that of being in control of a ton of steel and explosive fuel, defending his space on the highway.

But first, there is the driving test, which in the 1960's could not only be taken before the age of 17 years. In those days, there was no theory test – it was strictly practical.

"Mr. Worthington agreed. I fix his telly and he'll only charge me for the first two driving lessons – I'll get the others free. Reckons I'll pass with six lessons."

"Can you fix his telly?"

"Yeh, piece of cake. Prob'ly. Why do you think I'm doing a radio and TV repair apprenticeship you berk?"

"And you can use his car for the test?"

"Yeh. A Morris Thousand."

"Brilliant!"

"Yeh. Even the four lessons will make a big dent in my pay.– at a pound a lesson and that's nearly half my two pounds ten a week wages gone. I've got my first lesson Monday."

*

"I passed, I passed!"

"Yeh, and remember what the examiner said!"

"I'll never forget, never! He said – 'You're a good driver'".

"That's right. All he knows about you is your driving nothing else. You could be a normal person."

"Yeh – that's the first compliment anyone has ever given me. Ever. All those driving tips that Bob gave me when I was out in the car with him, they were really good. The examiner said my progressive braking was remarkable for a first time driver!"

"What's progressive braking? I thought the point of braking was *not* to make progress?"

"Stop jossing about! It's just gradually increasing the brake pressure so as not to lock the front wheels."

"Oh. And you passed in a Moggi Thou too! You didn't even crunch the gearbox."

"Yeh it was brilliant! Absolutely bloody brilliant! I'm going to buy a car. How much do you reckon I'll get one for? Fifty quid?"

"You'll prob'ly get something for that, maybe less, but Deer Leap Garage will be too pricey."

"Yeh, I guess so. What do you think then?

"Check the Gazette on Friday or Saturday. You might even see one for sale round the estates."

"Worth a look, but fifty quid! I'm not selling my radios."

"Those radios are scrap, old now, nobody'd want them anyway."

"Yeh, but I'll cut down on ciggies for a start, that'll save a few bob."

"Don't forget insurance, and tax too – you'll need all that. MOT too."

"Yeh, I'll never afford a car new enough to avoid the MOT. At least I'll be able to fix it up myself - learning about engines an' stuff with at Boxmoor, and the motorbike, will come in really handy.

I'll need to get a toolkit for the car too – maybe Bob Tolhurst can help me."

"Could always drive without tax and insurance too. Loads do."

"No way, not now I've got my licence – had enough trouble with the motorbike. The rozzers would be on to me like a shot.

"What do you think Susan will say when she finds out you passed the test?"

"I don't care, but it'll probably be something cruel."

*

Passing his driving test was a critical episode in his life. At last he consciously realised that he could think for himself. His self-esteem took a huge leap forward.

*

After the first year of apprenticeship, which had been split between Perivale Government Training Centre and Southall Technical College, a realisation developed inside him that he was good at electronics and that electronics held a real future for him.

By this time, Susan had finished her secretarial course and moved to Oxford to work.

*

The Next Job

"That's it, I've had enough. That bugger Dave Hood has got right to me. Some manager he is – no wonder they call him Robin. Cheap labour, that's all the apprentices are."

"You've jacked it at Rediffusion then?"

"Yeh. I knew more when I was at Boxmoor, and I'm forgetting it all at Rediffusion. I've got a job down at Alban Audio & TV while I look for something better. Two wasted bloody years."

"Even when you get your trade they don't keep you on. I'm getting out now, not wasting any more time there. I spoke to Bob. He's going to keep a lookout for me, for a job. He said Thursdays is a good day."

"What happens Thursday?"

"Jobs day in the Daily Telegraph. A supplement he called it. He'll look out for me."

"A supplement? Tablets you mean?"

"Bloody hell, you're getting boring. It's about time *you* started thinking for yourself!"

"I only think for you. My questions make YOU think. That's why I'm here, why I've always been here."

*

His next job was at Shipton Communications, who built the first commercial telephone answering machine in the UK. It was leading edge technology and so expensive that only major companies could afford them. They also made auto-dialling machines for marketing companies.

With this move, Bob Tolhurst suggested that he should set up a regular savings account and put £5 a month aside for a rainy day.

The work at Shipton was much more interesting. They also built the EDAS electronic dialling machine which was to feature in a James Bond film.

It was to be more than a year before the Susan's brother made the most important move in the development of his career. During that period, his experience increased, and new equipment was being introduced almost daily as the worldwide industry of consumer electronics became established. His social skills were improving in leaps and bounds and then je took his next big step.

*

"That's brilliant!"

"Yeh – my first car. Ford Anglia 105E."

"Stupid looking back window."

"Yeh, someone said they designed it on a Friday."

"Well, the same bloke must have designed that other car as well then."

"What car?"

"Consul – a classic I think it's called. Maybe he only worked Fridays?"

"Don't be daft. At least it doesn't collect bird shit."

"That's a good point. How much room is there in the back seat?"

"Enough, but it'll be a tight squeeze."

"Not so bad when you're fitting together though!"

"Too right. Trouble is, it's only got two doors, so it's a fiddle to get into the back."

"You can always help her in."

"Shut up, is that all you think of? Still, beggars can't be choosers, though the estate model would be nice. I could stretch out then. Four speed gearbox too, brilliant. And the heater works!"

"You won't need that up on the Downs, you'll be generating your own heat."

"I bloody hope so. It's cost me all my savings! Anyway, Bob Tolhurst says he'll show me how to service it. Tune it too. Something about setting the tappets."

"Tappets? What're they?"

"Things which go up and down, opening the valves to let the petrol in, then the exhaust gas out. They're operated by push rods. Bob says I have to adjust the tappet clearance to make it efficient, and not rattle. I have to use a feeler gauge."

"That sounds interesting."

"Well, it's nothing to do with girls, alright?"

"OK, but it does sound technical – how do you know all that?"

-167-

"Bob's been telling me. It's easy – not half as complicated as radio either. It's a four-stroke engine, not two-stroke like lawnmower or go-kart engines."

"Strokes? What does that mean?"

"Not what you're thinking you dirty bugger! Basically, the oil is separate from the petrol. On a two stroke they're mixed together. The engine turns two revolutions for each power stroke - four piston movements. On a two-stroke, it's only one revolution. The engine cooling is different too. That's the simple explanation. Anyway, I'm driving it round to show to Peter tomorrow."

"Then I'm hoping that Susan Tarry will come for a drive with me on the weekend."

"You don't hang around!"

"No – I've waited so long for this car, I just want to get moving."

"Oh. It's too much for me. I think I'll go to sleep."

"Best thing for you. I thought I'd told you I can manage from now on."

"Just checking."

*

"What's up – you look almost happy?"

"Well, nothing's been happening, but today was good. Bob called me over and showed me the Telegraph supplement. Masses of jobs, and one that he thought might be good for me."

"Well, what did he say?"

"You were there."

"I was sleeping. As I told you this morning, I'll be doing more of that. You've got to watch out for *yourself* now."

"I thought you were sleeping?"

"Well, I do like to keep in touch, you know…"

"Make up your bloody mind!"

"I'm too busy being yours!"

"Ok, Ok. There's an advert in the Telegraph for a job at Marconi in St Albans. Bob thinks I should apply for it."

"What's the money like?"

"Don't know, but they're a big company. It's not an apprenticeship, so it's got to be better than Rediffusion. And it's local, no more traipsing into Greenford."

"Will you live at home?"

"I doubt it. I've got to write for an application form. And then there's an interview…"

*

"That was a rum weekend. What do you reckon about that Frank Whitbread bloke then?"

"What, apart from the fact that he's an ex-rozzer, Vice Squad, you mean? Well, Mother seems to like him. I wonder where she met him. I bet he's got some stories to tell!"

"Yeh, I'll bet. Brighton and Hove – there's always stuff there in the summer with Mods and Rockers going at each other. Other stuff too, queer stuff, they say."

"Reckon he's bent then?"

"What, as in queer?"

"No you berk, not that kind of vice. Bent as in – y'know – took bribes an' stuff."

"How am I supposed to know that?"

"Well just thinking. I reckon all coppers are bent."

"You do?"

"Stands to reason, they must get tempted, and not always dosh either. Favours, like. Prozzies an' stuff."

"I don't know about Frank, he seems decent enough. Top drawer bloke. I get on great with him. But yeh, you've got to be suspicious of coppers. And that fancy motorbike."

"What, the Velocette Venom? Fancy motorbikes don't make him straight. I'd love one like that. It's really his son's anyway. I reckon he just borrows it when his son wants the car. Does make you wonder whether he's bent though."

"Yeh, prob'ly that's it, just borrowing. Tell you what though, I reckon he's getting pissed off at South Park Gardens."

"Pissed off?"

"You can see he gets worked up at weekends when Susan's back from Oxford and gets everyone running around her, like she's some sort of queen. Yeh, he's like a taxi driver for Susan, running her everywhere."

"Do you think she's jealous, then?"

"Don't know, but I don't reckon he'll be around much longer. There's no room for both of them in South Park Gardens. It's a pity because Mother seems to like his company. He's good for her I reckon. And I get on well with him, too. He makes time to talk to me, treats me normal. He's got no time for Susan, though. He never stays over, either. At least, as far as I know."

*

After a drive in the car and a pub lunch, he and Cathy had returned to South Park Gardens. It was a sunny Sunday afternoon – it's strange how the best memories always seemed to be on sunny days – and there was no-one else at home in number 14.

Mother and Susan had gone to South Africa on holiday, and would be away for ten days or so.

Susan's brother had waited many years for this moment, and the assignation was no disappointment, unlike so many initiations of its kind. No doubt that had been many other such trysts that very afternoon, the world over.

That night, he was again in bed, accompanied only by invigorating new aromas. As he fell asleep, he relived the afternoon. That, at least, he had in common with almost all young men at that point in their lives.

"What was it like?"

"Brilliant, absolutely brilliant!"

"What happened then?"

"I'm not going into detail now, I'm knackered."

"Yeh, properly knackered, I'll bet. Tell me a little though, please?"

"What I will remember is this. She kind of trembled and moaned so hard I thought I was hurting her."

"Never."

"Yeh, and then she let out this huge moan and all sort of subsided. I couldn't hold back and then I was done for too."

"So she came?"

"Yes, I suppose so, though I'm no expert now, am I?"

"No, I suppose not. Not after one go."

"Two actually."

"Two? You're randy you are. Go on…"

"Well, she wasn't a virgin, that's for sure."

"How do you know?"

"She said 'You don't need to worry about getting me pregnant, I already am. Anyway, if I hadn't been, I would be now, that's a fact.'"

"Blimey, that makes you think."

"Yeh, for sure. Surprised me all right. I wouldn't have thought that of her."

"Why not?"

"Well, she's nice."

"So what? She hopped into your bed. Just because you weren't the first doesn't make anything different."

"Fair enough, you're right. Still, it was really nice."

"When are you seeing her again?"

"Don't know. Nothing fixed up yet."

"She still seeing the other bloke then is she?"

"I didn't ask and I don't want to know. I'll probably bump into her in the week and see how the land lies then. Anyway, I'm going to sleep now."

The day had its bad moment too. He remembered just before falling asleep.

"He's dead."

"Who's dead?"

"Tim."

"Oh, no. How come?"

"Been in hospital for ages. Some disease – TB I think Cathy said."

"Well, they'll have enough plates now."

"That's not very nice – he was a good pal and they were all really nice to me. They were poor, yet they shared what they had. I loved going there for tea."

"Sad."

"Yeh. What's TB?"

"Dunno, must be nasty though – it obviously kills people."

"That's what's worrying me - only sick people go to hospital. I hope I don't catch anything when I go for my operation next week. I'm scared stiff."

"At least it should fix your teeth."

"Maybe. If my front teeth grow properly, then maybe the others will lay off a bit on the bullying. Still, it sounds scary 'removing a piece of bone so your front teeth can descend properly', that's what the ortho-wotsit said. What are they going to do – use a saw? Bone is hard, I reckon they will definitely have to saw it. Ughh, I can't bear to think about it!"

"No, just a hammer and chisel, that's all, chip it out – slowly! I reckon you'll only be in agonising pain for two or three months."

"You bugger, lay off, don't be so cruel!"

"I'm just your imagination, remember."

"Some comfort you are!"

Another step to manhood had been taken, but now it was as a typical young man he was setting about building a life and career. With a car, a girlfriend and a good job, he was to all intents and purposes, normal at last.

Inside though, there were still scars and deeply-etched painful memories, many of which would persist for decades. His experiences and character left him with, in his own words 'a very direct way of speaking to people, which often makes them feel uncomfortable.' Also, as happened with the horse that the butcher had promised him many years before, he took people's words at face value and didn't understand people who told lies.

*

By now, Mother was in a well-settled routine, with work at TAM, occasional socialising with her friend, Mrs. Malet. They took summer holidays together at Margate and Eastbourne. Also they both belonged to the Womens' Institute, but beyond the events at the W.I. and her cinema visits, Valerie did little socialising.

*

"She really is a nasty piece of work! Every bloody Sunday evening she asks – orders – me, I should say, to run her back to Oxford. 'You are my brother, I expect you to run me back to Oxford.' No thanks, no petrol money, nothing. I pity the man who marries her."

"Cool down."

"Well, it's getting to be too much now. Listening to her go on and on about her life, her friends, all the way to Oxford. Never so much as a thank you."

"Well, just make yourself scarce on a Sunday evening. Go back early to Greenford."

"Yes, I think I'll have to do that. Keep out of the way."

*

Marconi

"Did you see her face?"

"Yeh, I thought she was going to explode."

"She didn't half go on about it, then I thought she'd choke on her toast too."

"Once she starts on about something, she doesn't half rant."

"Well, it must stick in her throat, finding out that you earn more than she does."

"I'm earning more than she earns doing the typing or whatever at her fancy secretary job. I wonder if she'll tell her friends?"

"Briony knows. And Diana. I already told them."

"They're bound to say something to her then."

"She'll probably tell them that I'm fibbing or stealing it."

"You reckon?"

"Yeh, stands to reason – she's been telling them for years that I'm mentally ill. She's mad that I'm earning more than her. She was so angry! It almost made me smile."

"Careful, you're not used to that."

"Shut up!"

*

Moving On and Up

Susan's brother had married Maureen in 1970. Susan had been a bridesmaid at their wedding – it was the way things were done within families.

Their home was a ground floor bedsit with a shared kitchen in a semi in Boxmoor Village, owned by an elderly couple from Harrow. Despite being in Boxmoor, there were no connections with the School, and they were happy. Maureen worked part-time at Woolworths.

They now travelled in a Ford Anglia van, and Susan's brother had his Radio Amateur licence to transmit in plain voice on VHF frequencies (for which no Morse Code test was necessary); his call sign was G8BAL. They had no possessions, just the van and a two metre ham radio (a Communicator) QQV-3-10. The radio was transportable in the van.

Since joining Marconi, the realisation that he was good at electronics had taken firm hold, and he decided to move on and become independent, a contract engineer.

*

Whilst working as a legal secretary in Oxford, Susan was living in digs during the week. Whilst in Oxford she met and eventually became engaged to Michael, a student at Keble College. Coincidentally, Michael's father also had been employed by BOAC.

Michael visited Berkhamsted regularly, and was doted on by Susan's mother. Michael was very intelligent, with a diffident personality and much in awe of Susan.

The Robinson family provided him with emotional and other support whilst he was a student and struggling to make ends meet. However, not all support was welcomed.

On the evening before Susan's marriage, Michael mentioned that he was going to change the oil in his car. Susan's brother chipped in with an offer to help. The offer was dismissed brusquely.

The following morning, before the wedding, Susan's brother suggested that Michael took the car out to check that the oil filter was correctly seated. The suggestion was dismissed with scorn, but when the car was driven away it left a pool of oil on the driveway, unnoticed and with disastrous consequences for the car engine.

*

The wedding was held in Keble College Chapel, and the wedding reception was held on the College premises in Spring of 1971. The Best Man was Keith Best who later became an MP and enjoyed notoriety including being jailed in 1987 for the fraudulent purchase of shares during the privatisation of British Telecom.

After the ceremony in a quiet corner of the quad, behind some aged pillars, passers-by glanced at the young man who was apparently muttering to himself.

"I need some time to think."

"What about – the dreaming spires?"

"No. No, not that. I've just had a shock. People inside keep asking me why I didn't give Susan away at the church. As Father is dead, I am the man of the family, and they say I should have given her away. But I didn't – John Watson gave her away. People think it's odd. I hadn't thought about it before. I remember when I was five and Father died, Aunty Muriel always reminded that I was the man of the house. I never really understood what it meant."

"Who's John Watson?"

"He's the Minister to Berkhamsted Free Church."

"Susan's church?"

"Yes, that's right. He's nothing to do with the family, at least not directly."

"Did Susan ask you to give her away?"

"No, and it just didn't occur to me. She obviously didn't want me to."

"Well, that's hardly a surprise is it?"

"Not really, but you would think that now I'm on an even keel and I've got a good job, that she would treat me normally. She is much more civil than she used to be – she doesn't call me all those horrible things any more - at least, not to my face."

"So, what do you say when people ask you about not giving her away, and why Watson did it?"

"I just said that I didn't know I had to. That's the truth, but it makes me feel stupid."

"What does Maureen say?"

"I haven't asked her yet. If anybody else asks me though, I'm going to say that I wasn't asked. That's the truth too."

"Nothing wrong with the truth. Cheer up, go have another glass of beer."

"There's no beer here – this is an Oxford College reception. They don't do beer."

"Oh."

"It's not only the giving her away either, it's the photographs."

"What photographs?"

"Exactly. The wedding photographs, I wasn't in them."

"Where were you then? They usually take them coming out of the church don't they?"

"Well, that's what Maureen and I did at our wedding. Probably Susan didn't want me in them. It's a wonder I was invited at all."

"Don't think that."

"Well, what should I think? It will never end will it?"

"What?"

"This thing Susan has about me – it will just go on and on until one of us dies or until I cut off contact completely."

"Would you do that?"

"I suppose not, she is my sister after all. It might upset Mum too. Things have improved – she doesn't insult me straight to my face, it just the way that she behaves that gets to me. I thought it had all passed by. Seems I was wrong. It will always be there – ultimately she only cares about herself. Even with Mum – I think it must only be about what would happen when Mum died."

"That's harsh."

"Yes, well, she is too."

"After today, she's got a husband to care about."

"True, but I wonder how he will take to it."

*

Over the next few years, Susan and Michael moved home on several occasions, and her brother (with his van) assisted with the removals. It was the natural thing to do, to help one's sister – that is the way it was in all normal, loving families.

*

Even today, tensions remain between Susan and her brother, and legal advice prevents me from writing, even tangentially, everything that has been said and written on both sides.

Time has not been a healer.

*

In Retrospect

By the time he was twenty two years old, life had stabilised for Susan's brother and he was able to play an active, normal part in society. Recovery from the original trauma (if that is what it was) was by now complete, and he had overcome the additional challenges that his long term special schooling had presented him with.

Looking back, we can now use the name 'Chris'.

Today, Chris knows that he is a dyslexic. His son also inherited the condition.

Dyslexia is a term embracing a range of learning disorders, all centred around difficulty with learning to read. Sometimes the word 'disability' is associated with it, but there are many who would claim it is only a disorder – some even consider it a gift. Neither is it an intellectual disability, but one of comprehension, based on the brain's difficulty in processing graphical symbols (i.e. letters).

Since first being recognised in 1881, research has developed three sub-types – auditory, visual and attentional, and it is estimated that between 5% and 10% of the population may be affected.

Symptoms vary, as do the degrees to which it may present, but difficulty in learning to read is central. Poor timekeeping is one fairly common aspect associated with dyslexics. Difficulties dealing with spatial relationships manifest themselves at play – for example clumsiness and difficulty with hand-eye-limb coordination as need in ball games. Mis-pronunciation and confusion of words are other symptoms.

There are numerous (at least eight) theories as to the causes of dyslexia, and one theory suggests that dyslexics have the facility to access a part of the brain that most people cannot (which is why some consider it a gift). This enhanced access confuses perception and dyslexia results.

Most unfortunately, children who had this disorder were usually classified as stupid, at least up until late in the 20th Century – Chris is a clear illustration of what could go wrong in this respect.

Cures

Dyslexia is notorious for the prevalence of proprietary 'cures' and quack stories. There are several approaches to 'correcting' the disorder. Some say that it is not correctional at all – it is about teaching dyslexic people how to use the senses they have to understand the language that the rest of the population uses in written form. There may be some validity in this view, as several researchers have noted that dyslexia incidence varies across language types, with image based languages such as Chinese and Kanji (written Japanese) being notable in this respect.

Today, school teachers are trained to recognise the symptoms – or at least to investigate further when a child has difficulty learning to read. Such a child will have the reasons explained and be taught techniques to help with reading, being recognised as having special educational needs. Self-esteem will be built up by teachers as confidence is important to making progress.

Child Abuse

Current UK definitions of what constitutes child abuse have widened considerably since the late 1940s and 1950s. The NSPCC 'Child Protection Factsheet' includes criteria such as providing a child with 'inappropriate clothing' as abusive. So, wearing a girl's green blazer to a boys' school would be abusive. However, with today's social services support that would be unlikely to occur.

The practice at Epping House Special School of letting the children run around unclothed is would clearly be seen as abusive under today's guidelines.

Family Finances

In the early 1990s, the British Airways staff newspaper carried a story which said that the company had a surplus in their pension fund and wanted to hear from any retired employee (or their spouse) who was in hardship. Uncle Frank saw the article. Susan applied and a small pension was arranged for Mother.

Chris was "not privy to the family's finances."

Mother and Father

Chris has no recollection of any signs of affection between his parents. That was not unusual for that generation. His sister enjoyed cuddles with both her parents, but he does not remember any physical contact, not even holding his parents hands when out walking.

Schooldays

Many years later, Susan told Chris about a reaction from Father which had upset her. When they were pupils at Edgerton School, Father would occasionally pick them up in the car. One Saturday lunchtime Father was waiting – he had been away for three weeks and Susan was excited to see him. She ran towards him expecting to be picked up and hugged, but he told her not to be 'so stupid' as it had been raining and his uniform overcoat was damp. The smallest things may be remembered years later, and we can never know the effect that they have.

Victoria Church of England First School

Situated in the heart of Berkhamsted, it is now modern in most respects, except perhaps the main building.

As its website describes it today:

"We have a strong family atmosphere at Victoria and children are welcomed from all faiths and none. Our aim is that all children learn well and achieve their full potential through a varied and creative curriculum and our excellent results were recognized by Ofsted (July 2009), when we were judged to be an outstanding school.

Victoria is also an Eco School, Healthy School and Fairtrade School and the children are encouraged and trained to take responsibility for their health and the environment. This and our affiliation to St. Peter's Church help to define the unique character of the school."

Mother's Illness – Home Truths

It is the way with most families, that as parents age and their children become adults, the parents highlight events and people in the history of the family, giving their children new insights; often, the new information and parental opinions change the perspectives of their children, now adult, with adult experiences. In effect, family history is, to an extent, restated in the oral tradition.

Of course, the memories on both sides are less than perfect anyway, and deteriorating. Given normal mental health, the most deeply seated and rigorously programmed memories remain essentially unchanged, though they may become more distant. Many older people find that as they reach late middle age, their pattern of dreaming changes, and they start dreaming about events earlier in their lives; less so than the events of yesterday of even last week.

The efficiency of our brains in storing new memories, declines as we age, and perhaps the change in dreaming patterns is part of a refresh routine, to ensure that our autonomic programmes and deep-seated memories are refreshed and re-solidified during this late life period of decline, with the ultimate purpose of maintaining life (and sanity) as long as possible, perhaps.

*

Chris saw his mother every couple of weeks or so, when he gained new perspectives on some of the events in his life and the happenings in Dell Field Close and South Park Gardens. Family history and events were, to a limited extent, revisited.

"You remember that girl who used to walk slowly past the house in South Park Gardens?"

"No, Mum. Who?"

"Well, that was Susan…erm…Susan Tarry was it?"

"Yes, Susan Tarry lived at the end of the road."

"Well, she walked past the house, going to the post box, often."

"So. I can't remember it, Mum."

"She always stopped outside our house when she passed."

"Why?"

"Because she was looking for you."

"How do you know that?"

"A woman can tell. She liked you, and she was always looking for you."

"I didn't know that."

"You just take it from me, I knew."

"Why didn't you say something to me?"

"We never really talked did we?"

"No, never. Anyway, I went out with Susan Tarry for a while."

"I didn't know you that you courted her."

"It wasn't anything as serious as that. Anyway, we didn't talk much did we, as you said?"

*

Most siblings argue and disagree, but was his sister's attitude unusually cruel? Certainly a clever and high-achieving first child can overshadow a second child unless parents take particular care to maintain balance; many such second children rebel. This was not the case with Chris. The problem of imbalance was, arguably, internalized. He was undoubtedly a clever but shy child and with the problem of dyslexia being unrecognised he was doubly challenged. Chris distinctly remembers three occasions with his Mother when he tried to discuss Susan's attitude towards him. His mother didn't wish to discuss the matter, but he believes that someone in the close family planted the seed of the idea in Susan's mind at a very early age.

Eventually, Mother's frailty increased to the point where she was unable properly to care for herself. She sold her flat and moved into a care home at Cobham, near to Susan.

Up until this time, Chris had seen his mother regularly but now she explained that she didn't want to see him again because of what Chris might think of what was done. Nevertheless he continued to visit her a couple of times a year. During one visit his mother seemed to want to unburden herself. With regard to family finances, Granny Somers-Vine had died a relatively wealthy woman, and Mother explained to Chris that 'prior to Granny dying she left specific instructions that Christopher be treated equally because he had been treated so unfairly as a child'.

In the event, these wishes, if accurately recalled by his mother, were not complied with.

Chris later obtained a copy of Granny Somers-Vine's will and says that it does not reflect her wishes as related to him by his Mother. He continues to believe that the Will was not signed when Granny was mentally capable, as she had "suffered from Parkinson's Disease for more than five years before the date of the will".

Although his mother no longer wished to see him, he did visit occasionally with his son and Amy, his granddaughter.

Mother's Death

Mother's death uncovered a few family secrets and stories.

Frank Williamson (Uncle Frank) spent some time with Susan's brother after the funeral talking about old times. He mentioned the night of the suicide attempt and how he'd driven Valerie to the

North Middlesex Hospital. On the drive home afterwards, he said, Valerie had told him that she had more feeling for her cats than for Chris.

Deep Memories

Even now, the sound of the letterbox rattling as the postman pushes the mail through causes Susan's brother to start – just a small pulse of adrenaline into the bloodstream. It is a completely autonomous reaction to the sound, taking him back over sixty years to his childhood.

Such are the effects of programming on a young, developing and relatively uncluttered brain. The reaction becomes hard-wired, the circuit defined for the life of the brain.

When he was in his mid-fifties he underwent counselling. His counsellor explored his early years in depth, and one session covered the 'green blazer'.

"So, let's be clear. All the other boys wore blue blazers."

"Yes."

"And your mother sent you to school in a green blazer?"

"Yes."

"Then it's clear. She didn't want you."

*

What did become clear, though, during conversations with family members, was that Aunty Sheila would willingly have taken Chris on as a surrogate son. Aunty Sheila's mother was Doris (one of Father's two sisters). Such informal arrangements were not unusual in the 1950s, but the possibility, apparently, was never then discussed. Perhaps it was easier for Mother to accept the diagnosis of the psychologists and not have to accept that Chris's difficulties might have arisen as a result of possible maternal shortcomings on her part.

Certainly, in retrospect, Chris would have welcomed adoption by Aunty Sheila. Sheila was to remain childless and eventually adopted a son.

*

Amateur Radio

When he was 21, Chris obtained a license to transmit. This was a restricted licence, meaning that he could only use Amateur VHF bands and technology for transmissions. VHF users worked exclusively in 'plain voice', so no practical Morse code test was required.

Many years later, 'Citizens' Band' radio was legalized in the UK, with no requirement for Morse Code ability. Transmitter power was limited to 5 watts. Though licences were simple to obtain, many users were unlicensed, and many illegal rigs were grossly exceeding the legal power output and being used for worldwide transmissions.

Even today, though technology has moved on, the Radio Amateur qualification maintains its high standards, and does not embrace Citizens' Band.

When Chris was first married and had a Ford Anglia van, he carried his VHF rig in the van.

Epping House Special School

The school was closed in July 1997.

Many of the boys from later generations than Chris, are still in touch with one another – it has an active set of student alumni on the 'Friends Reunited' website, almost a hundred members, many with interesting profiles.

Patrick Mackay was a patient at Epping House in the early 1960s. In 1975 he was sentenced to life imprisonment for three murders (having been charged with five). He has confessed to a total of eleven murders.

Beech House/St Augustine's Hospital

The hospital later gained notoriety in the 1970s when it was the subject of a committee of inquiry into malpractice and mismanagement. St Augustine's Hospital closed in 1993.

In 1980, Chris visited Beech House, to present them with a gift – an Electronic Mastermind, which he had designed for Invictor Plastics, of Leicester. Paddy, who had been a Charge Nurse at Beech House when Chris was a patient, told him that all the staff at the Unit thought that he was so severely disturbed that he would live his entire life in institutions.

Later, Dr. Turl told Chris that when parents visited their children at the Unit, he cited Chris as an example of one of the most severely disturbed children going on to design the Electronic Mastermind game, and that parents should be optimistic and not give up hope.

Boxmoor House Special School

R A Carrington (Ronald Alfred) enjoyed a distinguished career as an outstanding headmaster of the school, and was made and M.B.E in 1979. I have been unable to locate any corroboration that he had been a 'Desert Rat', and so the rumour that the pupils shared must remain as just that. Sadly, standards at the school eventually declined and Boxmoor House Special School was closed in 2005.

The closure followed the conviction of a female teacher for having sex with a pupil, and an investigation by the NSPCC. The teacher was jailed for six years. The Headmaster (a Mr. Pawson) and four teachers were suspended, and an internal enquiry was held. [Source: Hemel Gazette].

Subsequently, the school re-opened in 2010, catering for age groups 11-16. [source www.hemeltoday.co.uk]

As of November 2011, the school has an unofficial Friends Reunited website, with over 160 past pupils staying in touch.

*

The Drifters did indeed perform a brief rehearsal in the grounds of Boxmoor School. They became Cliff Richard's backing group in 1958.

In 1959, to avoid confusion with the American group of the same name, they changed their name to 'The Shadows'.

In 1985, during a visit to his mother's home, she pointed out a story in the Hemel Gazette which mentioned that the pupils and teachers at Boxmoor School had built a go-kart using a lawnmower engine. Chris bought a second-hand racing kart, and presented it to the school.

Religion

In 1978, at the age of 31 years old, Chris was working at John Hadland Laboratories, in Bovingdon, near Hemel Hempstead. He was working on the development of photographic processing equipment for Mirror Group Newspapers.

Another employee began to debate religion with him. This was the first time he had discussed the subject at length since that fateful, heated discussion with the Vicar in Victoria Park School when he was eight years old. Soon after, he became a Christian. He practises to this day.

However, John Hadland Laboratories was later to become infamous.

John Hadland Laboratories

In 1971, two employees of the company – Fred Biggs and Bob Egle – died in mysteries circumstances. Almost 70 other people suffered from mysterious sickness as the so-called 'Bovingdon Bug' swept through the company.

At this time, the firm was manufacturing infra-red lenses for military applications, using thallium bromide-iodide, and the strange illness was eventually found to have been caused by poisoning.

Late in 1971, Graham Young, a former employee, was arrested by police. Thallium and other toxic materials were found in his flat. He was convicted of the murders.

He is believed to have been responsible for at least one other death – that of his stepmother, Molly, in 1962. At his first trial, aged just 15, he had admitted administering poison to his father, sister and a friend. Following his conviction for attempted murder, he was detained in Broadmoor Hospital under the Mental Health Act, for a period of 15 years. Released after just nine years being deemed fully cured, he joined John Hadland Laboratories.

Young died in Parkhurst Prison in 1990, officially from a myocardial infarction. There is speculation, though, that it was neither a natural event nor self-induced.

Maladjustment

'Maladjusted' is a term that has largely been superseded in the UK, with such children often being referred to as 'children having emotional and behavioural needs'.

On the face of it, this would appear to be rather loose as a definition and to refer to all children.

The term 'maladjusted' is still widely used in the US, where its definition is distinct from that of 'seriously emotionally disturbed' children.

The Care and Education of Children with Special Needs

As the spectrum of child and adolescent emotional problems has been researched and analysed in much more detail since Chris was born, the provision of specialist care facilities has widened and deepened. New approaches have been developed and assessed, with varying degrees of success.

Genetically based problems such as Dyslexia, Dyspraxia, Autism and Asperger's Syndrome are now recognised, and although not all are treatable, all are manageable and 'sufferers' quality of life (and that of their families) is significantly 'better' than would otherwise have been the case. Early diagnosis and intervention of these conditions has considerably reduced the incidence of downstream problems.

Importantly, identification of non-genetically based (i.e. socially conditioned) problems has improved, and detection (e.g. by school teachers) and 'self-referral' systems such as Childline are increasingly effective.

From the novel approach of Homer Lane at the 'Little Commonwealth' in the early 20th Century, through to Epping House, ideas about the care and education of disturbed/maladjusted children evolved. More advanced concepts were developed and novel care, therapeutic and educational centres such as Brynmelyn (set up by Brendan McNutt in 1984) were established. Some of their radical approaches to helping normalise patients with self-harm and other problems which may drive criminality have come in for criticism in the parts of the popular press and with some politicians – 'holidays for hooligans' being one unfortunately lurid headline. Nevertheless, authorities whose intervention seeks to help these young people continue to appreciate the outcomes that the near one–to–one specialist carer ratios provide.

Other approaches and techniques have also been subject to opprobrium in the Press. For example, 'Pindown' as a technique for handling violent adolescents was conceived and eventually discredited, for very good reasons other than media commentary.

It would seem that the successful 'normalisation' of challenged youngsters and adolescents is, *a priori*, dependent on high staff : patient ratios, where trained adults act as non-judgemental friends and advisors to help patients uncover and understand the basis of their difficulties so that they can overcome the early programming which has manifested itself in antisocial or self-destructive behaviour. It is, perhaps, a mechanistic view of behaviour, but if the analysis and newer care models contribute towards recovery, then that has to be a good thing. All this, of course, has to be achieved within the economic constraints to which care policies are subject.

This is the most expensive way to treat these patients; it is also, arguably, the most effective. To arrive at an accurate cost/benefit analysis of such treatment must include a 'whole-life' cost of *not* treating these children and adolescents.

Electroconvulsive Therapy ('ECT')

This form of treatment is still in use today, and though it may seem barbaric, it does work in many cases. Protocols and equipment have been refined and it continues to play a role in the treatment of certain conditions today. Its use is usually recommended for cases of severe depression which has not responded to other treatment, and also for mania and catatonia.

Research continues in an effort to understand the way in which it works on the brain to alleviate these conditions.

Special People

Carl Jung

I have been unable to find any confirmation that Carl Jung visited the North Middlesex hospital during 1957/58. Chris's memory is clear on the matter and of the German accented English spoken by the consultant whom he met with and believes to have been Carl Jung.

The Unknown Girl

To this day, Chris remembers the strong feelings he felt, even as a ten year old boy, for the 'rabbit hutch girl' who was six years older than him.

Peter B

At Boxmoor, Peter B was regarded as clever, and attained an 'O' Level in Carpentry at Apsley Grammar. The other boys nicknamed him 'The Academic'.

He and Chris remained firm friends until about 1968, when Chris started dating Maureen, whose sister Angela, was by that time married to Peter.

Peter went to work in an electrical retailer and then on to make a career in the Army, Following the Army, he became a service engineer.

Diana

Diana Wrigley, one of Susan's close friends, had been a girlfriend of Chris's for a short time.

In later life, he discovered that Mr. and Mrs. Wrigley had taken a shine to him when he was at Boxmoor House School. At the time, though, his perception was so clouded by the belief that he was friendless and unloved, that he could not believe that anyone could like him.

Caroline

Caroline, (Vivienne's friend) who Chris fancied but had been warned off by Mrs. Tolhurst, had a problem with 'substance abuse' and that was the reason – unknown to Chris at the time – why Mrs. Tolhurst thought it a bad idea for him to become involved.

Bob Tolhurst

Chris stayed in touch with the Tolhursts until 2007 when Bob died. Chris read the eulogy at his funeral.

Briony

Chris and Briony are friends to this day, as are Briony and Susan.

Sid Coombes

Sid Coombes and Chris kept in touch for about fifteen years, until Chris was about twenty four. At that time Sid was working in Gloucestershire.

Neighbours and Friends

Valentine Moore

Val Moore was killed in 1969, at the age of 56. Vastly experienced, with over 15,000 hours of flight time, he was at the controls of a VC10 aeroplane, 5N-ABD, of Nigerian Airways, which crashed in fog whilst trying to land at Lagos Airport.

The cause of the accident has never been fully explained. His flying was variously noted by assessors as individualistic in some aspects, unorthodox and competent.

Susan

In her adult life Susan became a successful businesswoman. She has featured in press stories about events which some people might describe as 'lurid'. Her husband became a prominent government legal advisor.

http://www.5rb.com/case/carpenter-v-associated-newspapers-ltd/ (Retrieved October 2011)

http://lexisweb.co.uk/cases/2001/november/carpenter-v-associated-newspapers-ltd (Retrieved October 2011)

http://www.thelawyer.com/house-of-commons-lawyer-found-guilty-of-abusing-the-court-while-defending-his-wife/102368.article as reported by Naomi Rovnick (Retrieved September 2011)

Susan's Brother

Following a successful career, Chris retired from electronic engineering having achieved his ambition of owning an Aston Martin DBS V8.

He later developed an interest in photography and his technical skills led him to innovate in wedding photography.

With the use of gels on flash heads the obvious effect of flash is considerably reduced in photographs. He has developed other techniques which make his photographic settings and style unique for marriages in the New Forest area of Hampshire where he now lives.

On the personal side, he now has a son and two grandchildren. This book has cast his relationship with his son in a new light.

Chris has been formally diagnosed as being dyslexic, but he has displayed characteristics - both physical and emotional – which could be indicators of other conditions. These were most salient during his first twenty years and included, largely in his own words:

-   Social awkwardness
-   Disliking groups of people
-   Noise

- Physical clumsiness
- A bit obsessive, a bit of OCD,
- Inability to make friends
- Preferring things to people
- Difficulty coping with sudden change
- Anxiety

To me, as a layman with no medical qualifications, these characteristics might today be seen as indicative of 'Asperger's Syndrome/High Functioning Autism'.

The relationship with his sister and brother-in-law continues to be difficult, and in communication with me there have been some rather unpleasant statements made about him. Of course, this sort of antipathy in a family is by no means exceptional. However, in all the months I spent with Chris working on this book, I never once observed any vitriol or bitterness in him.

Chris has worked hard to improve his communication skills and is now an experienced and confident public speaker He is available to talk to small groups about his experiences.

In the first instance, please contact the Editor.
editor@ezeebooks.co.uk

*

Author's Notes

This is story of a boy growing up in a Middle England just starting to recover from the Second World War. People are damaged and Great Britain is being rebuilt.

It has been related by a 63 years-old man, recalling his damaged childhood, a childhood which was far from ideal. It is essentially factual, though some names have been changed and some memories may not be perfect.

The subject wanted to relate the essence of his formative years, and it has been a very emotional experience both for him and the author. It has caused ripples within his family and has re-defined his relationship with his son.

From the outset, we set out to make this non-judgemental. I sought to ensure that this was not perceived as a 'score-settling' work, though it is, inevitably, based on one person's recollections. Being judgemental would be inappropriate – definitions under the broad heading of child abuse have been extended and refined in the last sixty years. Likewise, childcare standards and practise have changed, both for parents and the relevant professions. These changes have been significant, and contemporary (that is, 21st Century) definitions have been included by way of comparison.

Was his treatment fair and reasonable, even half a century ago? I draw no conclusions here, but invite you to consider the facts.

He was also very insistent that this be an uplifting delivery for readers. Certainly, he became a successful professional engineer and is now an innovative wedding photographer having overcome the considerable obstacles he has faced. He is quite clear in his assertion that overcoming his difficulties was possible as a result of small, everyday kindnesses that certain people had shown him. How many of us remember the first time that someone enquired after our well-being? He does.

There are several such instances in the narrative, with a strong underlying implication for us all: small kindnesses add up, and what may seem to us as everyday insignificant acts and favours –

even words - can have profound and cumulative effects over a lifetime. Unfortunately, the converse is also true.

Besides these rare kindnesses, aspects of his schooling were very important in helping him surmount his difficulties, and hopefully, these will become apparent as his early life unfolds.

In his story, he is referred to as Susan's Brother. When I first met him at the start of this journey, almost the first words he said to me were "the book will be called Susan's Brother".

You, the reader, should be led to the reason by the writer's craft, but he has asked that I explain why, before we set out to draw you into his early life.

He was defined by his sister, Susan. As a boy, his mother always introduced him to other people as 'Susan's brother' and when speaking to other people she never referred to him by his given name.

The Programs
There were two statements which were repeated to the young child by his father:

"Boys can't have teddy bears – they're for girls - you'll grow up soft."
"Boys don't cry."

There are two statements which were repeated to the growing boy by his sister, from a very early age. They are remembered verbatim, to this day:

"You are fat and clumsy, you can't read or write, no-one will ever want you and you'll never get anywhere in life."
"I don't know why God is punishing me so. All I ever wanted was a good-looking brother who had a decent job, who could give me money and introduce me to nice boys; and look what I've got!"

James Marinero,
March 2012

References

'A Century of Psychiatry, Psychotherapy and Group Analysis', Ronald Sandison, Jessica Kingsley Publishers, 2001.

Children's' Homes:
http://www.sciencedirect.com/science/article/pii/S0140197198901750

'Child Protection Fact Sheet', NSPCC (2010).

Graham Young:
http://en.wikipedia.org/wiki/Graham_Young

http://www.watfordobserver.co.uk/nostalgia/crimelibrary/grahamyoung/thebovingdonpoisoner/

'Psychopath', Clarke and Penycate, Routledge & Keegan Paul, 1976

Hemel Gazette: www.hemeltoday.co.uk

'The Creation of Dangerous Violent Criminals', Lonnie H Athens, Univ. of Illinois, Reprint, 1992.

'The Student Voice Handbook: Bridging the Academic/practitioner Divide', Warren Kidd (Author, Editor), Gerry Czerniawski (Editor). Emerald Group Publishing Limited.

'Understanding Media: The Extensions of Man', Marshall McLuhan, 1st Ed. McGraw Hill, NY, 1964.

'Wild', Jay Griffths, Penguin Books, 2006.

Other sources include Childline and The Institute of Psychiatry (various documents and reports).

Please Review This Book

Thank you for taking the trouble to read the book. I do hope that you found it interesting and informative. I also hope that is has given you some valuable insight into how negative messages can have dire consequences for children – and the importance to them of simple kindnesses.

I'm still learning my craft as an author and that's why I need your help. It would be immensely helpful to me if you could write a review for this book and publish it on Amazon.

Writing a review is easy! Just mention:
- Why you bought the book
- The two biggest lessons/benefits you got from reading it (an example or quote would be great here)
- My writing style (conversational?) and whether it engaging.
- Was the book too short? Too long?
- Was the true story content backed up with research and interesting or relevant facts?
- Is there anything you did not like about the book?
- Any negatives about the book?
- How is this book similar to other books you have read on the subject?
- Just a sentence in summary

To write the review, go to my book page on amazon via the link
www.susansbrother.com/reviews
Scroll down to the reviews section and just write an honest review (good or bad) and give my book as many stars as you think it deserves.

Thank you in advance,
James